Questions for the MRCPCH Part 2 Written Examination

Nick Barnes BSc MBBS MRCPCH
Specialist Registrar Paediatrics
Department of Paediatrics
John Radcliffe Hospital
Oxford

Julian Forton MA MB BChir MRCPCH
Specialist Registrar and Clinical Research Fellow
Department of Paediatrics
John Radcliffe Hospital
Oxford

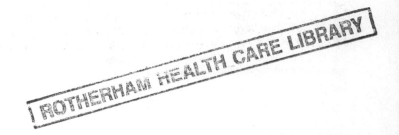

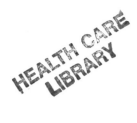

Telephone: 01565 752000

First edition 2004

ISBN: 1 904627 16 1

A catalogue record for this book is available from the British Library.
The information contained within this book was obtained by the authors from reliable sources. However, while every effort has been made to ensure its accuracy, no responsibility for loss, damage or injury occasioned to any person acting or refraining from action as a result of information contained herein can be accepted by the publisher or the authors.

PasTest Revision Books and Intensive Courses

PasTest has been established in the field of postgraduate medical education since 1972, providing revision books and intensive study courses for doctors preparing for their professional examinations. Books and courses are available for the following specialties:

MRCP Part 1 and Part 2, MRCPCH Part 1 and Part 2, MRCOG, DRCOG, MRCGP, MRCPsych, DCH, FRCA, MRCS and PLAB.

For further details contact:

PasTest Ltd, Freepost, Knutsford, Cheshire, WA16 7BR
Tel: 01565 752000   **Fax: 01565 650264**
Email: enquiries@pastest.co.uk   **Web site: www. pastest.co.uk**

Typeset by Saxon Graphics Ltd, Derby
Printed by Cambrian Printers, Aberystwyth

CONTENTS

INTRODUCTION

The written component of the Part 2 MRCPCH examination has historically consisted of three sections – long cases (grey cases), short cases (data interpretation) and clinical photographs. The examination has recently changed in format; the same material is now presented as longer cases integrating difficult differential diagnoses, data and photographs together to create a more in-depth clinical scenario.

The obvious advantage to this type of question is that the cases presented are more typical of everyday working practice. Understanding the expected progression of a disease, or the potential repercussions of certain interventions or omissions in treatment, is a part of medicine that is gained with experience rather than from straightforward texts. Children can become ill very quickly and their clinical condition often varies enormously *with time*. Continuous reassessment with expectant management is therefore of paramount importance and should be a daily routine. Using the *progression* of an ill child with time as the basis for a question, rather than presenting a snapshot in time, tests a more subtle knowledge of clinical paediatrics.

The questions in this book incorporate a clinical history with photographs, radiological investigations and data interpretation, and most involve several stages of decision making. Both general paediatrics and neonatology are covered. Each case-based question is accompanied by a comprehensive explanation and broad overview of the subject pertinent to the individual case.

Acknowledgements

We thank the Meningitis Research Foundation for permission to include the algorithm "Early Management of Meningococcal Disease in Children". We also thank the Consultant staff at the John Radcliffe Hospital, Oxford and at the Royal Berkshire Hospital, Reading for their advice in the preparation of this book.

GLOSSARY OF ABBREVIATIONS

ABPA	Allergic bronchopulmonary aspergillosis
ACE	Angiotensin converting enzyme
ACTH	Adrenocorticotrophic hormone
AER	Auditory evoked response
AIS	Androgen insensitivity syndrome
ALP	Alkaline phosphatase
ALT	Alanine transaminase
ANA	Anti-nuclear antibody
APTT	Activated partial thromboplastin time
ASB	Assisted support of breathing
ASD	Atrial septal defect
ASOT	Anti streptolysin-O-titre
AV	Atrioventricular
AVSD	Atrioventricular septal defect
BE	Base excess
BECTS	Benign epilepsy with centrotemporal spikes
CF	Cystic fibrosis
CK	Creatine kinase
CLD	Chronic lung disease
CMV	Cytomegalovirus
CMV	Continuous mandatory ventilation
CPAP	Continuous positive airway pressure
CRP	C-reactive protein
CSF	Cerebrospinal fluid
CT	Computed tomography
CTG	Cardiotocogram
DCT	Distal convoluted tubule

DHT	Dihydrotestosterone
DKA	Diabetic ketoacidosis
DMSA	Dimercaptosuccinic acid
DTPA	Diethylenetriaminepentaacetic acid
EBM	Expressed breast milk
EBV	Epstein-Barr virus
EMLSCS	Emergency lower segment caesarean section
ESR	Erythrocyte sedimentation rate
ETT	Endotracheal tube
FISH	Fluorescent *in-situ* hybridisation
GAL-1-PUT	Galactose-1-phosphate uridyl transferase
GORD	Gastro-oesophageal reflux disease
HCG	Human chorionic gonadotrophin
HDU	High dependency unit
HSV	Herpes simplex virus
IVC	Inferior vena cava
IVU	Intravenous urogram
LDH	Lactate dehydrogenase
LFT	Liver function test
LHRH	Luteinising hormone releasing hormone
LRTI	Lower respiratory tract infection
MAG3	Mercaptoacetyl triglycine
MCNS	Minimal change nephrotic syndrome
MCUG	Micturating cystourethrogram
MIBG	123-*m*-iodobenzylguanidine
MIH	Mullerian inhibitory hormone
MRI	Magnetic resonance imaging
NEC	Necrotising enterocolitis
NF	Neurofibromatosis
NG	Nasogastric
NPA	Nasopharyngeal aspirate
NVD	Normal vaginal delivery
OI	Oxygenation index
PA	Pulmonary artery
PAPVD	Partial anomalous pulmonary venous drainage
PCP	*Pneumocystis carinii* pneumonia
PCR	Polymerase chain reaction
PDA	Patent ductus arterious
PEEP	Positive end expiratory pressure

PIE	Pulmonary interstitial emphysema
PT	Prothrombin time
PUJ	Pelvico-ureteric junction obstruction
PUVA	Psoralen with ultraviolet A light
RAA	Renin-angiotensin-aldosterone
RAST	Radioallergosorbent test
RDS	Respiratory distress syndrome
RR	Respiratory rate
RSV	Respiratory syncytial virus
SARS	Severe acute respiratory syndrome
SCID	Severe combined immunodeficiency disease
SGOT	Serum glutamate oxaloacetate transaminase (aka aspartate aminotransferase, AST)
SIADH	Syndrome of inappropriate antidiuretic hormone secretion
SIMV	Synchronised intermittent mandatory ventilation
SIPPV	Synchronised intermittent positive pressure
SLE	Systemic lupus erythematosus
SSNS	Steroid sensitive nephrotic syndrome
SVC	Superior vena cava
SVT	Supraventricular tachycardia
TGA	Transposition of the great arteries
UAC	Umbilical artery catheter
USS	Ultrasound scan
UTI	Urinary tract infection
UVC	Umbilical venous catheter
VSD	Ventricular septal defect
VUR	Vesicoureteric reflux
VZIG	Varicella zoster immune globulin

QUESTION I

An 11-month-old girl, born at term with no perinatal complications, was admitted to hospital with high swinging fever, tachycardia and pyuria. Height and weight were on the 3rd centile. Urine from suprapubic aspirate revealed > 100, 000 organisms and Escherichia coli was grown on urine culture. She was treated successfully with iv cefuroxime for 5 days. She was commenced on prophylactic trimethoprim prior to discharge and was extensively investigated over the next 3 months.

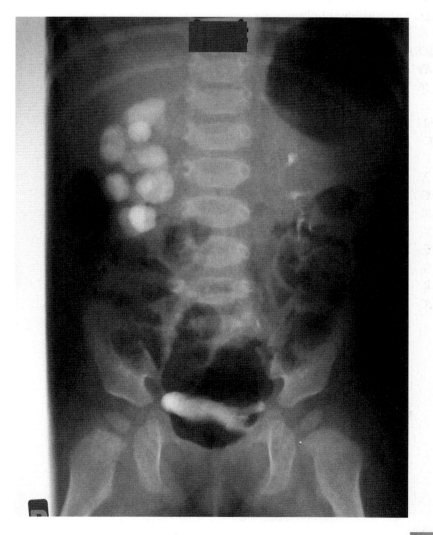

1.1 What investigation is this?

- ☐ A Micturating cystourethrogram
- ☐ B Indirect cystogram
- ☐ C Intravenous urogram
- ☐ D DMSA scan
- ☐ E DTPA scan
- ☐ F MAG3 scan (late views)

1.2 What is demonstrated?

- ☐ A Horseshoe kidney
- ☐ B Right-sided vesicoureteric reflux (VUR)
- ☐ C Left-sided ectopic kidney
- ☐ D Right-sided hydronephrosis
- ☐ E Right-sided duplication
- ☐ F Left-sided renal agenesis
- ☐ G Right-sided pyelonephritis

1.3 What is the likely pathology?

- ☐ A Right-sided grade 2 VUR
- ☐ B Right-sided grade 3 VUR
- ☐ C Right-sided grade 4 VUR
- ☐ D Right-sided pelvicoureteric junction obstruction
- ☐ E Left-sided pelvicoureteric junction obstruction
- ☐ F Posterior urethral valves
- ☐ G Right-sided renal scarring
- ☐ H Left-sided renal scarring

At 13 months of age she underwent the following procedure:

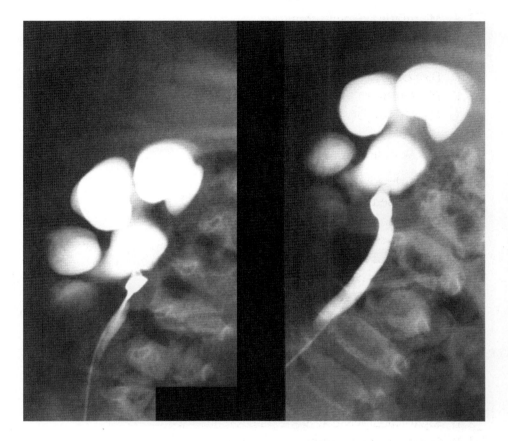

1.4   What is this intervention?

- [ ] A   Left-sided pyeloplasty
- [ ] B   Right-sided pyeloplasty
- [ ] C   Left nephrectomy
- [ ] D   Right nephrectomy
- [ ] E   Intravenous urogram
- [ ] F   Micturating cystourethrogram
- [ ] G   Reimplantation of left ureter
- [ ] H   Reimplantation of right ureter

Despite this intervention and ongoing trimethoprim prophylaxis she continued to have further urinary tract infections.

1.5 What does this investigation show?

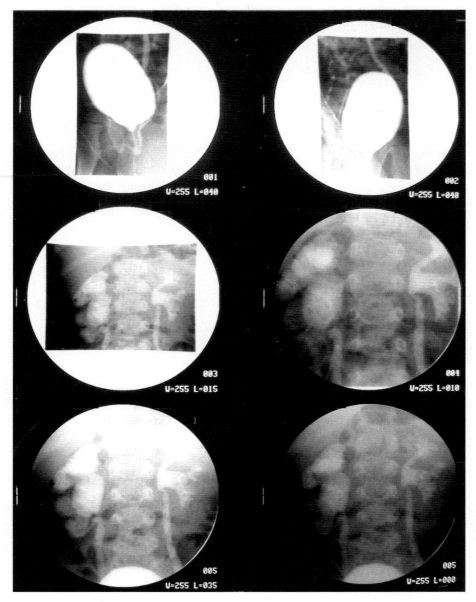

- ☐ A Bilateral grade 2 VUR
- ☐ B Bilateral grade 3 VUR
- ☐ C Bilateral grade 4 VUR
- ☐ D Posterior urethral valves
- ☐ E Bilateral calyceal clubbing with renal scarring
- ☐ F Bilateral pelvicoureteric junction obstruction

1.6 Which one intervention is indicated next?

. . . .

Following successful treatment, she became asymptomatic with no frank breakthrough urinary tract infections. She was lost to follow up for the next 4 years. The family moved back to the UK from New Zealand when she was 7 years of age, at which point her GP referred her to the paediatric clinic for review. Trimethoprim had been stopped at age 5 years.

1.7 How would you investigate her renal tract now?

- ☐ A BP, urinalysis, renal biochemistry, renal ultrasound, DMSA scan, MAG3 scan
- ☐ B BP, urinalysis, renal ultrasound, MCUG, DTPA scan, MAG3 scan
- ☐ C BP, urinalysis, renal biochemistry, renal ultrasound, MCUG, MAG3 scan
- ☐ D BP, urinalysis, DMSA scan
- ☐ E BP, urinalysis, renal ultrasound
- ☐ F BP, urinalysis, renal biochemistry, renal ultrasound, MCUG, DMSA scan
- ☐ G BP, urinalysis, renal biochemistry, renal ultrasound, DMSA scan, MAG3 scan

1.8 What does this investigation show?

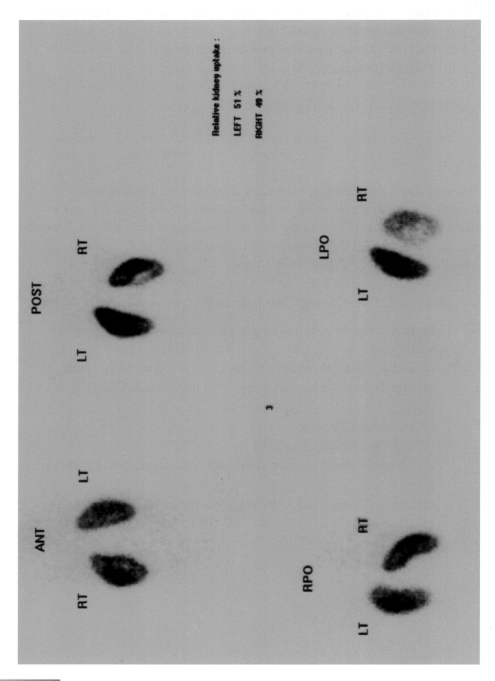

A Equal functional contribution from both kidneys, no evidence of scarring, prominent right renal pelvis

B Equal functional contribution from both kidneys, right-sided renal scarring

C Equal functional contribution from both kidneys, left-sided scarring

D Normal study

E Poor right-sided contribution, right-sided renal scarring

F Poor left-sided contribution, left-sided renal scarring

Consider the following investigations parts (a), (b), (c) and continue to question 1.9.

(a)

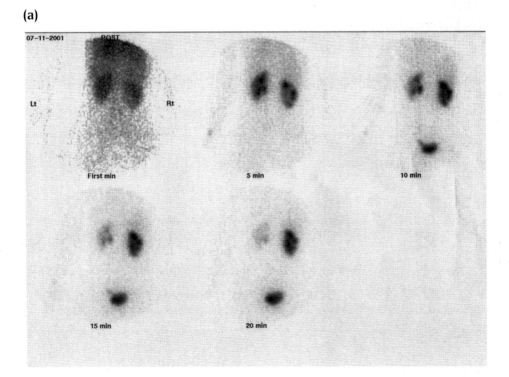

(b)

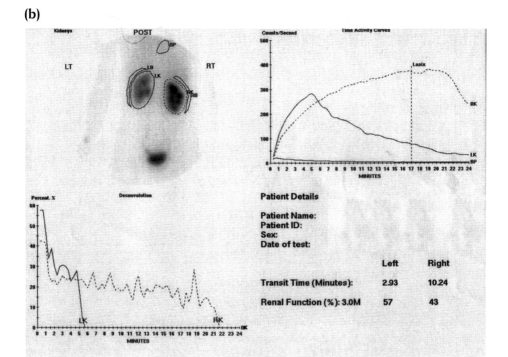

Patient Details

Patient Name:
Patient ID:
Sex:
Date of test:

	Left	Right
Transit Time (Minutes):	2.93	10.24
Renal Function (%): 3.0M	57	43

(c)

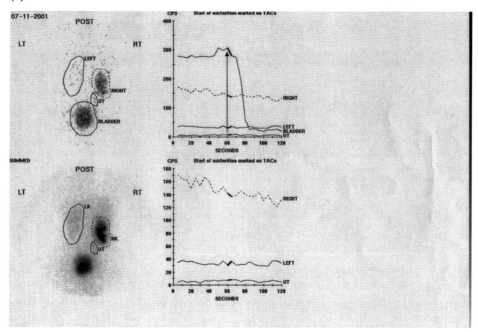

1.9 What does this investigation illustrate?

- ☐ A Decreased uptake left side
- ☐ B Decreased uptake right side
- ☐ C Normal left-sided renogram. Right side shows poor drainage, which improves with diuretic administration
- ☐ D Normal left-sided renogram. Right side shows poor drainage refractory to diuretic administration
- ☐ E Normal right-sided renogram. Left side shows poor drainage, which improves with diuretic administration
- ☐ F Normal right-sided renogram. Left side shows poor drainage refractory to diuretic administration

1.10 What does this represent clinically?

- ☐ A A baggy left-sided collecting system
- ☐ B A baggy right-sided collecting system
- ☐ C An obstructed left-sided collecting system
- ☐ D An obstructed right-sided collecting system
- ☐ E Right-sided renal scarring
- ☐ F Left-sided renal scarring

1.11 What is illustrated in part c of the investigation?

- ☐ A No VUR
- ☐ B Bilateral VUR
- ☐ C Scarring of right kidney
- ☐ D Scarring of left kidney
- ☐ E Reduced renal function bilaterally

Answers to Question 1 are on page 10

ANSWERS TO QUESTION 1

1.1 C   Intravenous urogram
1.2 D   Right-sided hydronephrosis
1.3 D   Right-sided pelvicoureteric junction obstruction
1.4 B   Right-sided pyeloplasty
1.5 C   Bilateral Grade 4 VUR
1.6   Bilateral reimplantation of ureters or endoscopic sub-mucosal Teflon injection
1.7 A   BP, urinalysis, renal biochemistry, renal ultrasound, DMSA scan, MAG3 scan
1.8 A   Equal functional contribution from both kidneys, no evidence of scarring, prominent right renal pelvis
1.9 C   Normal left-sided renogram. Right side shows poor drainage which improves with diuretic administration
1.10 B A baggy right-sided collecting system
1.11 A No VUR

Discussion

Pelvicoureteric obstruction may present with an abdominal mass or UTI. Most cases are detected prenatally. The majority of asymptomatic cases can be treated conservatively.

Indications for pyeloplasty include:

- Increasing hydronephrosis
- A drop in split function below 40%
- Symptoms (pain, recurrent UTI, haematuria, calculi)
- Bilateral pelvico-ureteric junction obstruction

Vesicoureteric reflux (VUR) is graded from 1 to 5:

1 Reflux into the lower ureter without dilatation
2 Reflux into the upper collecting system without dilatation
3 Reflux into dilated ureter with/without calyceal blunting
4 Reflux into a grossly dilated ureter with calyceal blunting
5 Reflux into a tortuous, dilated ureter with calyceal effacement

Grades 1 and 2 have a high rate of spontaneous resolution. Grade 3 carries a 50% chance of requiring surgical treatment. Grades 4 and 5 have a low rate of spontaneous resolution and early surgical intervention is indicated.

Investigation of urinary tract infection in children

Following a confirmed UTI, all children require further investigation. The aim of investigation is to identify children with risk factors for developing renal parenchymal damage.

The major risk factors are:

- anatomical abnormalities that predispose to infection, eg obstruction, renal calculi
- VUR.

Children under the age of 5 years are treated with prophylactic antibiotics until VUR is excluded. If they have documented VUR they will be treated with prophylactic antibiotics until the age of 5 years, after which point VUR is unlikely to cause further scarring even if still present.

There is no universal consensus as to which investigations are indicated in children with confirmed UTIs. The guidelines below are generally accepted:

In all children under the age of 1:

- USS of renal tract defines anatomy
- MCUG excludes VUR
- DMSA scan indicates if renal scarring is already present.

In all children aged 1–5 years of age:

- USS of renal tract defines anatomy
- DMSA scan indicates if renal scarring is already present
- Direct (MCUG) or indirect (MAG3 or DTPA) cystography for assessment of VUR is indicated if:
    - the DMSA scan shows scarring
    - the UTI was suggestive of acute pyelonephritis with systemic signs
    - there are recurrent infections
    - there is a family history of VUR

In all children over 5 years of age:

- USS of renal tract defines anatomy
- DMSA scan if:
    - the USS is abnormal

- the UTI was suggestive of acute pyelonephritis
- there are recurrent infections
- there is a family history of VUR

(If VUR is still present after the age of 5, it is unlikely to cause further scarring, so cystography in this age group is not routinely indicated.)

Summary of investigations

Abdominal X-ray will help exclude opaque calculi and spina bifida.

DMSA (dimercaptosuccinic acid) scan has the greatest specificity and sensitivity for detecting renal scarring and defining renal split function.

DTPA (diethylene triamine pentacetic acid) and **MAG 3 renograms** are dynamic isotope scans which can be used to define scarring and split function, provide information about obstruction and assess VUR indirectly without the need for catheterisation.

IVU (intravenous urogram) will demonstrate PUJ obstruction or obstruction from renal calculi. It is useful in defining abnormal renal anatomy eg horseshoe kidney, duplex kidneys and ectopic ureters.

MCUG (micturating cystourethrogram) is the standard investigation for defining VUR and defining urethral anatomy.

Renal ultrasound defines anatomy of kidneys, ureters and bladder.

QUESTION 2

A 9-year-old girl is referred to outpatients with a 1-week history of cramping abdominal pain, anorexia and constipation. She has not passed a stool for 6 days. There is no history of vomiting or urinary symptoms. She has been weak and lethargic for the last month, and has frequently complained of sore legs. Her parents say that she has been bullied recently at school and they are concerned that some of her symptoms may be psychosomatic. In the clinic she is unable to stand or lift her head up straight, and so is admitted to the ward for investigation. Further symptomatic enquiry is largely unremarkable, although her parents say she has had great difficulty in climbing the stairs over the last week and they have resorted to carrying her. They also think she has lost weight over the last month.

Neonatal history was unremarkable. She had a splenectomy aged 7 following a road traffic accident and is on long-term prophylactic penicillin. She has had Pneumovax® and is up to date with the standard immunisation programme. Her father has ischaemic heart disease and mild hyperlipidaemia for which he has been prescribed simvastatin. Her mother is well. The family live on a farm, and her 11-year-old brother has previously been successfully treated for infection with Trichinella spiralis, which manifest as abdominal pain and diarrhoea. The whole family was screened at that time and only her brother was found to be infected.

On examination, her temperature is 37.5°C, pulse 84, blood pressure 95/60 and respiratory rate 18. She has a hoarse voice. She is unable to lift her head up off the pillow and has difficulty sitting upright. Cardiovascular and respiratory examination is unremarkable. Abdominal examination is difficult as she is nervous and upset, but she is centrally tender with a mobile mass palpable in the left iliac fossa. There is no rebound or guarding. Bowel sounds are normal. On neurological examination, her cranial nerves are intact. Peripheral examination reveals mildly reduced four-limb tone more marked proximally. Her arms and legs are tender on palpation. Arm abduction and elbow flexion is MRC grade 3/5 bilaterally. Other arm movements are normal. Biceps reflex is reduced bilaterally, though triceps and supinator reflexes are normal. Hip flexion is grade 4/5 bilaterally, with otherwise normal leg active movements. Knee jerks are reduced bilaterally; ankle jerks are both normal and she has flexor plantar reflexes bilaterally. She has great difficulty in standing to walk from her bed unaided. Gower's sign is positive. Neck examination is normal.

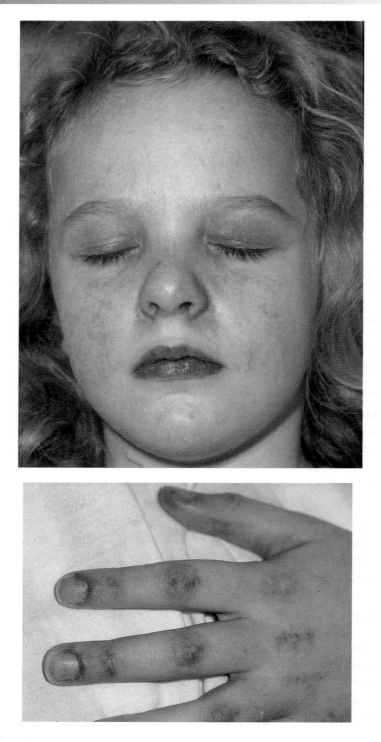

Her GP has already carried out the following investigations:

Haemoglobin: 9.8 g/dl
Platelets: 449×10^9/litre
White cell count: 4.4×10^9/litre
ESR: 32 mm/h
Sodium: 138 mmol/litre
Potassium: 4.2 mmol/litre
Urea: 2.9 mmol/litre
Creatinine: 55 μmol/litre

2.1 What is the most likely diagnosis?

- [ ] A Systemic lupus erythematosus
- [ ] B Acne rosacea
- [ ] C Drug-induced lupus erythematosus
- [ ] D Guillain–Barré syndrome
- [ ] E Photosensitive dermatitis
- [ ] F *Streptobacillus moniliformis* infection
- [ ] G Endocarditis
- [ ] H Dermatomyositis
- [ ] I Tinea facei
- [ ] J Myasthenia gravis
- [ ] K Poliomyelitis
- [ ] L Acute influenza B infection
- [ ] M Psoriasis
- [ ] N Hyperthyroidism
- [ ] O Ingestion of father's medication
- [ ] P Erysipelas
- [ ] Q Seborrhoeic dermatitis
- [ ] R Becker muscular dystrophy
- [ ] S Hypothyroidism

2.2 What do her hands show?

- [ ] A Garrod's pads
- [ ] B Psoriatic plaques
- [ ] C Photosensitive dermatitis
- [ ] D Janeway lesions
- [ ] E Rheumatoid nodules

☐ F Severe eczema with lichenification
☐ G Lupus-related skin vasculitis
☐ H Peripheral acne rosacea
☐ I Gottren's papules
☐ J *Streptobacillus moniliformis* systemic infection
☐ K Osler's nodes
☐ L Hypersensitivity reaction
☐ M Tinea capitis

✓ **2.3 Which THREE of these tests are likely to be most helpful in confirming the diagnosis?**

☐ A Wood's light examination
☐ B Anti-ribonucleoprotein antibody
☐ C Anti-La antibody
☐ D Rheumatoid factor
☐ E Echocardiogram
☐ F Anti-double-stranded DNA antibody
☐ G Skin swab
☐ H Anti-nuclear antibody
☐ I Anti-smooth muscle antibody
☐ J CSF protein
☐ K Viral titres
☐ L Anti-histone antibody
☐ M Blood culture
☐ N Anti-Ro antibody
☐ O Stool culture
☐ P Creatine kinase
☐ Q Skin scrapings
☐ R Thyroid function testing

Whilst on the ward awaiting assessment she becomes breathless soon after having a drink. Her mother had just gone out to the toilet at that point, and so isn't certain exactly what happened. You are urgently called to the ward to review her. On examination her temperature is 37.8°C, heart rate 105, respiratory rate 30 and oxygen saturations 91% in air. On chest auscultation, she has crepitations in her right mid-zone. Her abdomen is diffusely tender, but there is no rebound or guarding, and bowel sounds are audible.

Her mother asks you what you think has happened.

2.4 **What is the most likely explanation for her respiratory problems?**

☐ A Acute pneumonitis
☐ B Right-sided pneumothorax
☐ C Inhaled foreign body
☐ D Liquid aspiration
☐ E Pneumonia
☐ F Pancreatitis with a reactive pleural effusion
☐ G Lung vasculitis secondary to lupus erythematosus
☐ H Pleural effusion secondary to lupus erythematosus
☐ I *T. spiralis* lung infiltration
☐ J Early pulmonary fibrosis

2.5 **With this diagnosis in mind, which ONE daily test would now be useful to guide further management?**

☐ A Spirometry
☐ B Chest X-ray
☐ C Pulse oximetry oxygen saturation
☐ D Peripheral blood white cell count
☐ E Videofluoroscopy
☐ F Amylase
☐ G Total IgE

2.6 **How do you account for her abdominal pain?**

☐ A Constipation
☐ B Volvulus
☐ C Intussusception
☐ D Appendicitis
☐ E Lower lobe pneumonia
☐ F Pancreatitis
☐ G Secondary to *T. spiralis* infection

2.7 Once stabilized, which ONE of the following is the most appropriate treatment option for her underlying condition?

- [ ] A Intravenous antibiotics
- [ ] B Prednisolone and intravenous antibiotics
- [ ] C Oral antibiotics
- [ ] D Topical prednisolone
- [ ] E Stop prophylactic penicillin and start alternative
- [ ] F Plasmapheresis
- [ ] G Oral prednisolone
- [ ] H Referral to paediatric cardiology centre
- [ ] I Cold tar preparation topically
- [ ] J PUVA

Answers to Question 2 are on page 20

ANSWERS TO QUESTION 2

2.1 H Dermatomyositis

2.2 I Gottren's papules

2.3 F Anti-double-stranded DNA antibody

    H Anti-nuclear antibody

    P Creatine kinase

2.4 D Liquid aspiration

2.5 A Spirometry

2.6 A Constipation

2.7 G Oral prednisolone

Discussion

Juvenile dermatomyositis is a systemic vasculopathy resulting in focal myositis and characteristic cutaneous findings. Periorbital violaceous erythema, Gottren's papules and a rash over the extensor surfaces are classical. Skin involvement may precede frank myositis, and the onset of proximal muscle weakness may be insidious, difficult to recognise and eventually manifest as difficulty in standing, combing hair and climbing stairs. Gower's sign is commonly positive.

Hoarseness, choking and aspiration may occur as a result of involvement of upper airway muscle, and constipation, abdominal pain, diarrhoea and infarction as a result of impaired gastrointestinal smooth muscle function. Cardiac conduction defects, dilated cardiomyopathy, hepatosplenomegaly, ocular involvement and seizures have also been reported. Calcinosis affects up to 20% at presentation, diminishing with aggressive steroid therapy.

At diagnosis CK, SGOT and LDH are all elevated, and ANA is positive (speckled pattern) in 60%. ESR may be normal or elevated, with a normocytic anaemia and lymphopenia commonplace. ESR and CK can be used to monitor response to treatment.

A paediatric rheumatologist should supervise management. If clinical uncertainty regarding the diagnosis exists, EMG and muscle biopsy are usually confirmatory; diagnostic yield from these investigations can be increased with the use of MRI to localize the active site of disease. Steroids are the mainstay of treatment, pulsed methylprednisolone being reserved for those with severe disease (respiratory and palatal involvement) at presentation. Methotrexate and cyclophosphamide have been used in cases unresponsive to steroid therapy. Cyclophosphamide may precipitate a haemorrhagic cystitis, though the risk of such is reduced with the concomitant administration of mesna. It may also result in irreversible infertility. Dysphagia associated with this condition may necessitate tube feeding, and, in rare cases of respiratory failure, tracheostomy and ventilation may be required. Physiotherapy and sunscreen are important aspects of treatment.

Mortality is currently 3%, and the period of active symptoms typically 18 months with aggressive immunosuppressive therapy. Long-term morbidity in children is under evaluation.

QUESTION 3

Consider the following list of diagnoses:

List A

A   Transposition of the great arteries
B   Tricuspid atresia
C   Partial anomalous pulmonary venous drainage (PAPVD)
D   Secundum ASD
E   VSD with left-to-right shunt
F   VSD with Eisenmenger's syndrome
G   Tetralogy of Fallot with right-to-left shunt
H   Tetralogy of Fallot
I   Truncus arteriosus
J   Patent ductus arteriosus
K   Aortic stenosis
L   Pulmonary stenosis
M   AV malformation
N   Peripheral pulmonary stenosis
O   None of the above

For each set of cardiac catheter measurements below, choose the most appropriate diagnosis from List A.

3.1 Age 9

	Oxygen saturation (%)	Blood pressure (mmHg) (systolic/diastolic)
SVC	88	
IVC	65	
Right atrium	83	
Right ventricle	83	30/6
Pulmonary artery	83	30/20
Pulmonary vein	96	
Left atrium	90	
Left ventricle	90	90/6
Aorta	90	90/60

3.2 Infancy

	Oxygen saturation (%)	Blood pressure (mmHg) (systolic/diastolic)
SVC	65	
IVC	65	
Right atrium	83	6
Right ventricle	83	35/6
Pulmonary artery	83	35/15
Left atrium	96	6
Left ventricle	96	90/6
Aorta	96	90/60

3.3 Age 8

	Oxygen saturation (%)	Blood pressure (mmHg) (systolic/diastolic)
SVC	65	
IVC	63	
Right atrium	64	4
Right ventricle	64	30/4
Pulmonary artery	64	30/10
Left atrium	96	7
Left ventricle	96	100/7
Aorta	96	100/60

3.4 Age 8 months

	Oxygen saturation (%)	Blood pressure (mmHg) (systolic/diastolic)
SVC		
IVC		
Right atrium	64	3
Right ventricle	80	40/6
Pulmonary artery	80	40/20
Left atrium	96	6
Left ventricle	96	100/6
Aorta	96	100/60

3.5 Age 10

	Oxygen saturation (%)	Blood pressure (mmHg) (systolic/diastolic)
SVC		
IVC		
Right atrium	65	3
Right ventricle	65	95/6
Pulmonary artery	65	95/60
Left atrium	96	6
Left ventricle	80	95/6
Aorta	80	95/60

3.6 Age 12

Age 12	Oxygen saturation (%)	Blood pressure (mmHg) (systolic/diastolic)
SVC		
IVC		
Right atrium	60	4
Right ventricle	60	95/6
Pulmonary artery	60	35/4
Left atrium	96	6
Left ventricle	84	95/6
Aorta	84	95/55

3.7 Day One

	Oxygen saturation (%)	Blood pressure (mmHg) (systolic/diastolic)
Right atrium	60	7
Right ventricle		
Pulmonary artery	88	88/40
Pulmonary vein	96	
Left atrium	88	6
Left ventricle	88	90/7
Aorta	88	90/50

3.8 1 week of age

	Oxygen saturation (%)	Blood pressure (mmHg) (systolic/diastolic)
Right atrium	60	4
Right ventricle	80	90/6
Pulmonary artery	80	90/50
Left atrium	96	6
Left ventricle	80	90/6
Aorta	80	90/50

3.9 Age 24 hours

	Oxygen saturation (%)	Blood pressure (mmHg) (systolic/diastolic)
Right atrium	50	6
Right ventricle	50	80/6
Pulmonary artery	96	50/8
Left atrium	96	
Left ventricle	96	
Aorta	50	80/60

Answers to Question 3 are on page 26

ANSWERS TO QUESTION 3

3.1 C   Partial anomalous pulmonary venous drainage
3.2 D   Secundum ASD
3.3 O   None of the above (normal cardiac catheter)
3.4 E   VSD with left-to-right shunt
3.5 F   VSD with Eisenmenger's syndrome
3.6 G   Tetralogy of Fallot with right-to-left shunt
3.7 B   Tricuspid atresia
3.8 I   Truncus arteriosus
3.9 A   Transposition of the great arteries

Discussion

Cardiac catheterisation can be used as both a diagnostic and therapeutic procedure. From a diagnostic perspective, pressure gradients and oxygen saturation measurements can give detailed information about the size of shunts, pressure gradients across valves and the degree of pulmonary or systemic vascular resistance.

Cardiac catheter data is given as saturations and systolic and diastolic pressures in the different compartments of the heart and circulation. It is important to know the normal values (Question 3.3). An approach to analysis is first to concentrate on the oxygen saturations. Start at the IVC/SVC and work round to the right atrium, right ventricle and pulmonary artery. The blood entering the right side of the heart is usually deoxygenated with saturations around 60–70%.

For blood moving through the right-sided circulation, a step up in oxygen saturations of > 5% suggests there is a left-to-right shunt at that level:

> 5% difference in IVC compared with SVC	PAPVD	(3.1)
> 5% rise in oxygen saturations in the right atrium	ASD	(3.2)
> 5% rise in oxygen saturations in the right ventricle	VSD	(3.4)
> 5% rise in oxygen saturations in the pulmonary artery	PDA	

Similarly, for blood moving through the left-sided circulation, a step down in oxygen saturations of 5% suggests that there is a right-to-left shunt at that level:

> 5% drop in oxygen saturations in the left atrium	ASD	(3.1, 3.7)
> 5% drop in oxygen saturations in the left ventricle	VSD	(3.5, 3.6)

In addition to the above findings, for there to be a significant intracardiac right-to-left shunt, right sided pressures will be equal or higher than left sided pressures (see ventricular systolic pressures in Questions 3.5, 3.6).

A large pressure gradient across a valve suggests stenosis. Questions 3.5 and 3.6 both demonstrate a right-to-left shunt at ventricular level with high right ventricular pressures. The two cases can be differentiated by the pulmonary artery pressures. In Question 3.5, the PA pressures are also raised, indicating that the right ventricular outflow tract is not obstructed, and pulmonary vascular resistance has increased secondary to increased blood flow through an uncorrected large left-to-right shunt. This situation is very undesirable as increased pulmonary vascular resistance will become irreversible with time (Eisenmenger syndrome). Large intracardiac left-to-right shunts that cannot be repaired immediately can be managed with pulmonary artery banding to protect the pulmonary vasculature from high blood flow and inevitable pulmonary hypertension. In Question 3.6, the pulmonary artery pressure is low despite high right ventricular pressures, and this suggests that the right ventricular outflow is obstructed. In context, this could represent tetralogy of Fallot with a right-to-left shunt at ventricular level, but would also fit for a child with a large VSD who has had pulmonary artery banding that has now become too restrictive as he has grown.

Question 3.7 demonstrates a right-to-left shunt at atrial level – saturations and pressures are equal in both aorta and pulmonary artery. This fits with tricuspid atresia without VSD where blood from the right atrium reaches the pulmonary artery exclusively via the left atrium, left ventricle, aorta and patent ductus.

In Question 3.8, both ventricular systolic pressures are equal and aortic and PA pressures are equal. This would fit with truncus arteriosus. Univentricular heart without obstructed outflow to either vessel would also fit with this pattern.

QUESTION 4

Consider the following list of disorders:

A Ornithine transcarbamylase deficiency
B Medium chain acyl-CoA dehydrogenase deficiency
C Glycogen storage disorder type 1a
D Glycogen storage disorder type 1b
E Glycogen storage disorder type 2
F Glycogen storage disorder type 3
G Gaucher's disease
H Refsum's disease
I Canavan's disease
J Mucopolysaccharidosis
K MERRF syndrome
L MELAS syndrome
M Galactosaemia
N Nesidioblastosis
O Ketotic hypoglycaemia
P Hereditary fructose intolerance
Q Beckwith–Weidemann syndrome
R Exogenous insulin administration
S Organic acidaemia
T Growth hormone deficiency

✓ Case I

A 5-month-old child is brought to A&E with a 3-day history of cough and runny nose associated with mild fever. His parents report that he has been otherwise well with normal growth and development. He is small with a weight on the 0.8th centile, but this has increased recently with the introduction of a variety of solid foods, which he seems to tolerate well. He has not been feeding properly for 48 hours and has deteriorated steadily over the day with vomiting and increasing lethargy. He is now unrousable; pulse 130, BP 100/60, respiratory rate 60, oxygen saturations 100% in air. Respiratory and cardiovascular examination is otherwise unremarkable. He has a palpable liver at 5 cm below the costal margin but no splenomegaly or palpable lymphadenopathy. He is jaundiced.

Initial investigations are:

Blood gas (venous):   pH 7.05; pCO_2 3.4; pO_2 6; HCO_3^- 14; BE −11
Lactate: 2.0 mmol/litre
Blood glucose: unrecordable
Urine MC+S: unremarkable
Urine reducing sugars: positive

4.1   **From the list of disorders which is the most likely diagnosis?**

. . . .

✓**Case 2**

A 2-month-old Asian girl of consanguineous parents is brought to A&E, unrousable with unrecordable blood sugar levels. Systems examination is otherwise unremarkable. Weight and head circumference are on the 50th centile. Bloods are taken prior to resuscitation with 2 ml/kg 10% dextrose followed by an iv infusion (equivalent to 5 mg/kg per minute). Her blood glucose level after 1 hour of treatment is 5 mmol/l.
   Initial investigations are:

Blood glucose: 0.4 mmol/litre
Blood gas (venous):   pH 7.1; pCO_2 3.4; pO_2 6; HCO_3^- 16; BE −9
Lactate and liver function tests: unremarkable
Ammonia: 45 μmol/litre
Urinary reducing sugars: negative
Urinary ketones: negative
C peptide: absent
Organic acid profile: raised levels of dicarboxylic acids
Insulin, growth hormone, cortisol
and thyroid hormone levels: pending

4.2   **From the list of disorders, which is the most likely diagnosis?**

. . . .

Case 3

A 7-day-old boy, born at term without perinatal complications, is admitted to hospital with increasing lethargy, vomiting and tachypnoea. There has been no history of fever and on examination he is afebrile. He is unrousable. Pulse is 150, respiratory rate 50 and BP 80/40. Examination is otherwise unremarkable with no signs of infection or cardiac disease. He is resuscitated appropriately and commenced on iv antibiotics.

    Tests showed:

Blood glucose:	1.7 mmol/litre
Blood gas (venous):	pH 7.28; pCO_2 4.5; pO_2 6; HCO_3^- 21; BE −4
Lactate and liver function tests:	unremarkable
Ammonia:	1515 μmol/litre
Urinary ketones:	positive
C- peptide:	absent
Insulin, growth hormone, cortisol and thyroid hormone levels:	pending

4.3   Which TWO of the following tests would be most useful in confirming the correct diagnosis?

☐ A Urine dipstick for reducing sugars
☐ B Insulin
☐ C C peptide
☐ D Free fatty acids
☐ E Serum lactate
☐ F Plasma glutamine, aspartic acid and alanine
☐ G Plasma organic acids and plasma amino acids
☐ H Urinary levels of orotic acid
☐ I Uric acid
☐ J Lipid profile
☐ K Plasma acyl carnitine levels

4.4   From the list of disorders which is the most likely diagnosis?

. . . .

Case 4

A 5-day-old boy, born at term without perinatal complications, is admitted to hospital with poor feeding, vomiting and increasing lethargy. There has been no history of fever and on examination he is afebrile. On examination pulse is 140, respiratory rate 60 and BP 100/40. He is unrousable and hypotonic. Examination is otherwise unremarkable. Blood tests are taken and he is resuscitated with intravenous fluid and glucose. Despite volume resuscitation and a serum glucose maintained above 4, his condition does not improve. He is treated for sepsis and meningitis. Lumbar puncture is deferred.

   Initial investigations are:

Blood glucose:	1.2 mmol/litre
Blood gas (venous):	pH 6.9; pCO_2 4.3; pO_2 6.3; HCO_3^- 11; BE −14
Lactate:	2.1 mmol/litre
Liver function tests:	unremarkable
Coagulation studies:	unremarkable
Electrolytes:	unremarkable
ESR:	4 mm/hour
CRP:	12g/l
Ammonia:	540 μmol/litre
Urinary ketones:	positive
Urinary reducing sugars:	negative
Urinary MC+S:	unremarkable

4.5 Which one of the following would be most useful in confirming the correct diagnosis?

☐ A Urine dipstick for reducing sugars
☐ B Insulin
☐ C C peptide
☐ D Free fatty acids
☐ E Serum lactate
☐ F Plasma glutamine, aspartic acid and alanine
☐ G Plasma organic acids and plasma amino acids
☐ H Urinary levels of orotic acid
☐ I Uric acid
☐ J Lipid profile
☐ K Plasma acyl carnitine levels

4.6 From the list of disorders which is the most likely diagnosis?

. . . .

Case 5

A 3-month-old boy is admitted to hospital with a 2-day history of coryzal symptoms with worsening lethargy over the last 24 hours. Height and weight are below the 0.8th centile. On examination he is unrousable. Pulse is 140, respiratory rate 60, saturations 100% in air, BP 90/50. He has a protuberant abdomen with massive hepatomegaly palpable 6 cm below the costal margin. There is no splenomegaly or peripheral lymphadenopathy. Examination is otherwise unremarkable. Blood tests are taken and he is resuscitated with intravenous fluid and glucose, and commenced on iv antibiotics.

Initial investigations are:

Blood glucose:	0.3 mmol/litre
Blood gas (venous):	pH 7.05; pCO_2 6; pO_2 6; HCO_3^- 16; BE -9
Lactate:	14.1 mmol/litre
Haemoglobin:	11.0 g/dl
White cell count:	4.0×10^9 litre
Neutrophils:	$\underline{0.2} \times 10^9$ litre
Platelets:	160×10^9 litre
The serum is reported as lipaemic	
Liver function tests:	unremarkable
Ammonia:	30 μmol/litre
Na:	$\underline{130}$ mmol/litre
K:	4.3 mmol/litre
Urea:	2.4 mmol/litre
Creatinine:	34 μmol/litre
Chloride:	102 mmol/litre
PT, APTT:	unremarkable
Urinary reducing sugars:	negative
Urinary MC+S:	unremarkable

4.7 From the list of disorders which is the most likely diagnosis?

. . . .

4.8 Which TWO tests would be most useful in supporting your diagnosis?

☐ A Urine dipstick for reducing sugars
☐ B Insulin
☐ C C peptide
☐ D Free fatty acids
☐ E Serum lactate
☐ F Plasma glutamine, aspartic acid and alanine
☐ G Plasma organic acids and plasma amino acids
☐ H Urinary levels of orotic acid
☐ I Uric acid
☐ J Lipid profile
☐ K Plasma acyl carnitine levels

4.9 How is the definitive diagnosis made?

. . . .

Case 6

A 9-day-old boy is admitted to hospital with hypoglycaemia and lethargy. On examination, he is unrousable, his pulse is thready, rate 170, respiratory rate 60 and blood pressure 50/30. Cardiovascular examination is otherwise normal. He is afebrile and there are no frank signs of infection. Examination is otherwise unremarkable. Blood tests are taken and he is resuscitated with intravenous fluid and glucose and commenced on iv antibiotics.

Initial investigations are:

Glucose:	2.7 mmol/litre
Blood gas:	(venous) pH 7.3; pCO_2 4.5: pO_2 6; HCO_3^- 23; BE −3
Haemoglobin:	13.2 g/dl
White cell count:	4.2×10^9/litre
Platelets:	300×10^9/litre
Na:	124 mmol/litre
K:	7.2 mmol/litre (not haemolysed)
Urea:	4.6 mmol/litre
Creatinine:	40 μmol/litre

4.10 What is the most likely diagnosis and what test will confirm this diagnosis?

. . . .

. . . .

4.11 What further treatment is necessary?

. . . .

Answers to Question 4 are on page 36

ANSWERS TO QUESTION 4

4.1 P Hereditary fructose intolerance
4.2 B Medium chain acyl-CoA dehydrogenase deficiency
4.3 G Plasma organic acids and plasma amino acids
        H Urinary levels of orotic acid
4.4 A Ornithine transcarbamylase deficiency
4.5 G Plasma organic acids and plasma amino acids
4.6 S Organic acidaemia
4.7 D Glycogen storage disorder type 1b
4.8 I Uric acid
        J Lipid profile
4.9   Liver biopsy
4.10   21α-Hydroxylase deficiency; 17-OH progesterone levels
4.11   Steroid replacement (hydrocortisone and fludrocortisone)

Discussion

Hypoglycaemia with acidosis is a rare presentation. In the first 1 month of life, most cases will be due to severe infection or a cardiac pathology. However, hypoglycaemia with acidosis should always trigger consideration of metabolic disease as an underlying aetiology.

Glucose levels are reduced by insulin and increased by the counter-regulatory hormones glucagon, growth hormone, cortisol and adrenaline. Under increased stress, these counter-regulatory hormones maintain levels of glucose by increasing breakdown first of hepatic glycogen by glycolysis, then fat breakdown through beta oxidation, which also produces ketones, and finally in the later stages by protein breakdown via the urea cycle.

In hyperinsulinaemic hypoglycaemia (macrosomia from gestational diabetes, Beckwith–Wiedemann syndrome, nesidioblastosis, pancreatic adenoma), glucose is pushed into fat stores and causes a persistent hypoglycaemia requiring large amounts of glucose iv to maintain plasma glucose levels (generally 10–15 mg/kg per minute compared to normal rates of 4–6 mg/kg per minute). Because fat breakdown is inhibited, ketones are absent in hyperinsulinaemic states. If insulin levels are found to be raised and C peptide is present, the source of insulin is exogenous and this is suggestive of Munchausen-by-proxy.

(Fatty acid oxidation defects also present with hypoglycaemia and acidosis. Because beta-oxidation is blocked by the enzyme defect, ketones are absent. Acyl carnitine is the intermediate, which accumulates in medium chain acyl-CoA dehydrogenase deficiency, the most common of the fatty acid oxidation defects. These children may also have a dicarboxylic organic aciduria. ✓

Deficiencies in enzymes involved in gluconeogenesis and glycolysis in the liver will cause a block in the metabolic pathway, with resultant accumulation of an intermediate metabolite. Classic galactosaemia results from deficiency in galactose-1-phosphate uridyl transferase (GAL-I-PUT) and commonly presents in the first month of life. Lactose from milk contains galactose and glucose. Without the transferase enzyme, galactose-1-phosphate cannot be metabolised, accumulates in the liver and inhibits normal breakdown of glycogen, causing hypoglycaemia. The metabolite is toxic to the kidney, liver and brain. These infants often present with hypoglycaemia, acidosis, hepatomegaly and jaundice, and are at increased risk of *Escherichia coli* sepsis. A preliminary diagnosis can be made by documenting a non-glucose reducing sugar in the urine (Clinistix® positive, Glucostix® negative).

✲ Hereditary fructose intolerance results from a deficiency in fructose-1,6-bisphosphonate aldolase (aldolase B), the enzyme that incorporates fructose into the glycolytic pathway. Children with this disorder are perfectly well until exposed to fructose-containing foods, which usually happens when solids are first introduced. Rapid accumulation of fructose-1,6-bisphosphonate on exposure to fructose is toxic to the liver, with clinical manifestations resembling galactosaemia. Again, hypoglycaemia and acidosis is accompanied by hepatomegaly, jaundice and non-glucose reducing sugars in the urine.

Glycogen storage disorders are the group of diseases caused by deficiencies in the enzymes involved in the synthesis or breakdown of glycogen. Those principally affecting liver enzymes generally present with hypoglycaemia and hepatomegaly. Patients with type 1 glycogen storage disorder (Von Gierke's disease) have a deficiency of glucose-6-phosphatase with consequent reduced conversion of glycogen to glucose. Glycogen accumulates in the liver causing massive hepatomegaly. The intermediate glucose-6-phosphate is redirected to produce lactate. The classic presentation is between 3 and 4 months of age with hypoglycaemia, profound lactic acidosis and massive hepatomegaly. LFTs may be normal.

Triglycerides are markedly elevated causing a milky lipaemia. Uric acid levels may also be elevated. Children with type 1b glycogen storage disease have neutropenia and impaired neutrophil function in addition to the findings listed above. In the presence of lipaemia, assays for serum sodium are artificially low, as seen in case 5.

Amino acid catabolism involves the production of ammonia, which is fed into the urea cycle. Here useful metabolites are produced that are channelled into the Kreb cycle for oxidative phosphorylation, and urea is produced as the non-toxic nitrogenous waste product. Ammonia itself is highly toxic to the central nervous system. Urea cycle defects are caused by deficiencies in the enzymes of the urea cycle. In the neonatal period the accumulation of ammonia occurs over the first few days of protein feeding and principally affects brain function with rapidly progressing lethargy and coma. These infants are often misdiagnosed as having sepsis. There may be few clues aside from the raised ammonia levels to suggest a metabolic disorder, as these disorders rarely cause acidosis. Ammonia levels are massively elevated (> 1000 μmol/litre). Liver function tests are usually normal. Most of the urea cycle defects have raised plasma levels of a specific amino acid which aids diagnosis. The most common urea cycle defect is caused by ornithine transcarbamylase deficiency (X-linked). This has no specific amino acid elevation in the plasma but orotic acid levels in the urine are raised.

A deficiency in enzymes involved in the catabolism of amino acids will result in the accumulation of intermediates in the amino acid degradation pathway feeding the urea cycle. These children will have a specific aminoacidaemia. If the intermediate that accumulates is acidic, then the disease is termed an organic acidaemia and will usually present with profound metabolic acidosis and hypoglycaemia with an unexplained anion gap. Ammonia levels will be moderately raised (generally up to 1000 μmol/litre). In the most severe forms, children will appear normal at birth but develop poor feeding, vomiting, lethargy and coma within the first week of life as they are exposed to milk proteins.

Preliminary metabolic investigation

For preliminary metabolic investigation into hypoglycaemia and acidosis, the following diagnostic framework can be applied to most clinical situations.

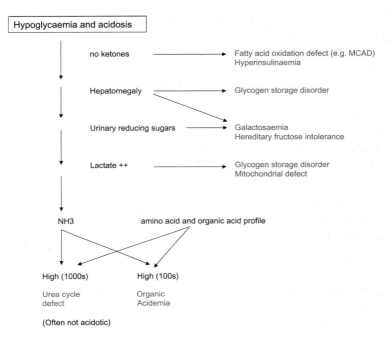

Hypoglycaemia and acidosis

no ketones → Fatty acid oxidation defect (e.g. MCAD)
Hyperinsulinaemia

Hepatomegaly → Glycogen storage disorder

Urinary reducing sugars → Galactosaemia
Hereditary fructose intolerance

Lactate ++ → Glycogen storage disorder
Mitochondrial defect

NH3   amino acid and organic acid profile

High (1000s)   High (100s)

Urea cycle   Organic
defect   Acidemia

(Often not acidotic)

Preliminary metabolic investigation: summary of investigations and associated disorders.

Urinary reducing sugars
- Galactosaemia
- Hereditary fructose intolerance

Absence of ketones
- Hyperinsulinaemic hypoglycaemia (nesidioblastosis, Beckwith–Wiedemann syndrome, infant of diabetic mother, pancreatic adenoma)
- Fatty acid oxidation defects

Hepatomegaly
- Galactosaemia
- Hereditary fructose intolerance
- Glycogen storage disorder

Hepatomegaly and jaundice
- Galactosaemia
- Hereditary fructose intolerance

Raised lactate
- Glycogen storage disorder
- Mitochondrial defect

Raised ammonia
- Urea cycle defect (1000's)
- Organic acidaemia (100's)
- May be raised as result of liver dysfunction

Organic acidaemia
- Organic acidaemia
- Fatty acid oxidation defect (dicarboxylic acidaemia)

Aminoacidaemia
- Aminoacidopathy
- Urea cycle defect

C peptide
- Exogenous insulin administration

✓QUESTION 5

A 6-day-old boy is admitted to hospital in January with a short history of poor feeding, lethargy and jitteriness. He was born at term by normal vaginal delivery, birthweight 3.5 kg, with good Apgar scores. There were no perinatal risk factors for sepsis. First day check was unremarkable and he was discharged home on day 2. There is no significant family history. He has one older sister age 3.

On examination he is lethargic, pyrexial, tachycardic with a pulse of 150, normotensive, and has oxygen saturations of 88% in air, 96% in 5 litres/min mask oxygen. Capillary refill time is 4 seconds. Cardiovascular examination is otherwise normal. His respiratory rate is 60, though air entry is good bilaterally with minimal recession. His abdomen is non-tender, with a 3 cm hepatomegaly. ENT examination is unremarkable. He has a left exudative conjunctivitis. He has no rash.

A partial septic screen is performed, which he tolerates well. He is given mask oxygen, a bolus of 10 ml/kg 0.9% saline, commenced on maintenance iv fluids, iv cefotaxime and ampicillin, and observed on HDU. A self-limiting apnoea lasting 10 s is observed on the ward.

Initial investigations are:

Haemoglobin:	17.5 g/dl
White cell count:	5.1 × 10^9/litre (N 2.3, L 2.2)
Platelets:	73 × 10^9/litre
CRP:	17 g/litre
Glucose:	5.4 mmol/litre
Sodium:	130 mmol/litre
Potassium:	3.7 mmol/litre
Urea:	4.5 mmol/litre
Creatinine:	42 μmol/litre
Urinalysis:	leukocytes −, nitrites −, protein +, blood trace, ketones +, SG 1025, glucose −
Lumbar puncture:	deferred

Chest X-ray on admission

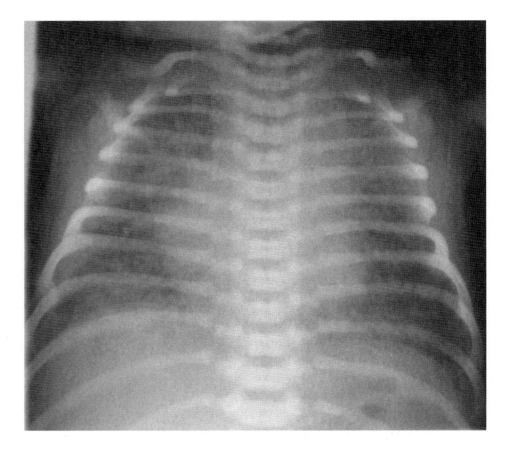

5.1 **What are the five diagnoses most compatible with the above findings?**

☐ A Group B streptococcal sepsis
☐ B *Escherichia coli* sepsis
☐ C EBV infection
☐ D CMV infection
☐ E Herpes simplex infection
☐ F Respiratory syncytial virus infection
☐ G HIV infection
☐ H Systemic candidal infection
☐ I Chlamydia infection
☐ J Necrotising enterocolitis
☐ K Rotavirus infection
☐ L Intracranial haemorrhage
☐ M Urinary tract infection
☐ N 21-α-hydroxylase deficiency
☐ O Transposition of the great arteries
☐ P Pulmonary stenosis
☐ Q Large VSD

On reassessment 4 hours after admission he is more lethargic, more tachycardic with a pulse of 180 and has developed an increasing oxygen requirement. Sats 95% in 50% headbox oxygen. He has 6 cm hepatomegaly.

Further results now show:

AST:	7305 IU/litre
Alkaline phosphatase:	207 IU/litre
Total bilirubin:	25 μmol/litre
PT:	> 200 seconds
APPT:	> 200 seconds

5.2   What is the diagnosis?

- ☐ A   Group B streptococcal sepsis
- ☐ B   *E. Coli* sepsis
- ☐ C   EBV infection
- ☐ D   CMV infection
- ☐ E   Herpes simplex infection
- ☐ F   Respiratory syncytial virus infection
- ☐ G   HIV infection
- ☐ H   Systemic candidal infection
- ☐ I   Chlamydia infection
- ☐ J   Necrotising enterocolitis
- ☐ K   Rotavirus infection
- ☐ L   Intracranial haemorrhage
- ☐ M   Urinary tract infection
- ☐ N   21-α-hydroxylase deficiency
- ☐ O   Transposition of the great arteries
- ☐ P   Pulmonary stenosis
- ☐ Q   Large VSD

Answers to Question 5 are on page 46

ANSWERS TO QUESTION 5

5.1 A Group B streptococcal sepsis
    B *Escherichia coli* sepsis
    E Herpes simplex infection
    F Respiratory syncytial virus infection
    Q Large VSD
5.2 E Herpes simplex infection

Discussion

This child is febrile and unwell with diffuse patchy shadowing on chest X-ray. The commonest bacterial cause of this scenario is Group B streptococcal pneumonia/sepsis. *E. coli* sepsis is also a frequent cause of bacterial sepsis in this age group. The portal of entry is nearly always the urinary tract. Since in this case urinalysis is negative, and there is a respiratory focus, *E. coli* sepsis is less likely. However, *E. coli* can be acquired from swallowing infected amniotic fluid in utero or through transplacental spread and must be considered in the differential diagnosis nevertheless. RSV bronchiolitis could explain all the findings in the initial assessment and is a well-known cause of apnoea in young infants. The conjunctivitis should alert you to the possibility of HSV infection or chlamydia infection. This child is too young for chlamydial infection, which usually occurs around week 4 of life, but these X-ray changes would fit with the interstitial pattern seen in chlamydial pneumonia. An infant with a congenital cyanotic heart defect that is duct-dependent may present in the first days of life when the duct closes. However, in this case, the infant's oxygen saturations responded to oxygen indicating that he is unlikely to have congenital cyanotic heart disease. A large VSD, however, may cause sufficient left-to-right shunting for a child to present with cardiac failure even at this early age.

Disseminated herpes simplex infection must always be considered in the differential diagnosis for sepsis in the first 14 days of life. HSV pneumonitis is well described in the first 7 days of life, may be the sole presenting feature of HSV infection, and is rarely considered in the differential diagnosis for neonatal respiratory distress. It rapidly progresses to disseminated HSV disease. This child developed multi-organ failure and died on day 27 of life. HSV type-2 was isolated from his eye swab and CSF.

Up to 80% of women with genital herpes have no lesions at the time of delivery and no known history of genital herpes, and are therefore not identified to receive preventative obstetric management, nor expectant paediatric input. Although the individual risk of HSV transmission in this group is very small, > 70% of cases of neonatal HSV arise from this population of mothers. It follows therefore that, although a history of HSV in the mother is certainly helpful, its absence does not eliminate the risk of vertical transmission. (Cutaneous manifestations of neonatal HSV infection (skin, eye, mouth) require immediate iv aciclovir, as without treatment there is a 70% risk of developing disseminated HSV infection or encephalitis. Disseminated neonatal HSV infection usually occurs in the first 14 days of life, and typically presents with non-specific signs such as poor feeding, lethargy and fever. There are no cutaneous manifestations in 50% of cases. Dramatically elevated liver function tests and coagulopathy are common, and helpful in making an early diagnosis. Mortality is of the order of 70% even with treatment.

QUESTION 6

A 12-year-old girl with cystic fibrosis experiences an increase in her chest symptoms. She does not have a chronic cough but in the last 3 weeks has been coughing daily. She saw her GP about 2 weeks ago, was noted to be wheezy and was given a 5-day course of 30 mg prednisolone once daily, together with advice to use a salbutamol inhaler as required. This seemed to help her chest symptoms, but in the last few days she has been coughing again. The family have two dogs. They live in an old house and have recently had an extension built. There is no family history of atopy, foreign travel or known contact with tuberculosis. Her current medications are pancreatic enzyme replacement capsules, vitamins A and D, ursodeoxycholic acid and omeprazole.

On examination she has finger clubbing. Respiratory rate is 24 and air entry is moderately good bilaterally. She is hyperinflated and has bilateral polyphonic wheeze and crepitations audible all over her chest. Oxygen saturations are 96% in air. Heart sounds are normal with no murmurs. She is apyrexial. She has lost weight since she was last seen in clinic 6 weeks ago.

Lung function results are as follows:

12 months ago

```
INDEX     PRED     MEAS     %
FVC       1.94     2.29    118
FEV1      1.74     1.88    108
FEV1%       89       82     92
PEF        255      256    100
F2575     2.22     1.76     79


INTERPRETATION OF TEST RESULTS:


COMMENTS:
```

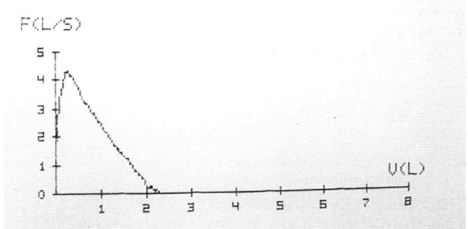

Current lung function

```
                                   !-- Normal --!
              Base %Pr Post %Pr %Chg Min Pred Max
FEV1          1.11  65            1.42 1.71 2.05 L
FVC           1.46  74            1.68 1.99 2.35 L
PEF            170  63             205  274  343 L/M
FEV1/FVC        77  89              85   86   88 %
```

Flow Volume Loop

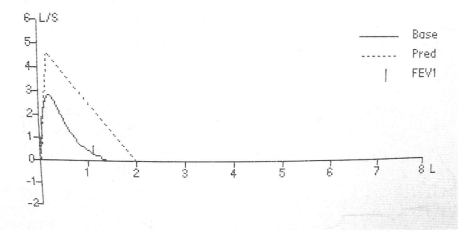

6.1 **Which THREE conclusions can be drawn from the results of lung function testing?**

☐ A   She has a restrictive lung disorder
☐ B   Her lung function is better now than it was 12 months ago
☐ C   She has normal lung function
☐ D   No specific conclusions can be drawn as she has not made a good enough effort for the results to be reliable
☐ E   No comparison can be made between the two studies as she is currently unwell
☐ F   She has a degree of small airways obstruction
☐ G   Her lung function is worse now compared with 1 year ago
☐ H   She has a mixed obstructive-restrictive picture
☐ I   She has asthma
☐ J   She has cystic fibrosis related bronchial hyperreactivity

In view of her persisting symptoms further investigations are undertaken. The results are as follows:

Haemoglobin:	14.7 g/dl
White cell count:	13.5×10^9/litre
Neutrophils:	6.4×10^9/litre
Lymphocytes:	3.7×10^9/litre
Monocytes:	0.3×10^9/litre
Eosinophils:	3.4×10^9/litre
Platelets:	212×10^9/litre
Cough swab:	Upper respiratory flora only (culture report at 5 days)

She is given a 2-week course of ciprofloxacin but fails to improve. A salbutamol inhaler is similarly of no benefit. A chest X-ray is requested.

12 months ago

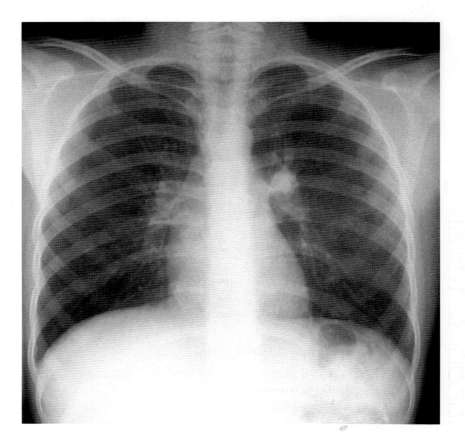

Current chest X-ray

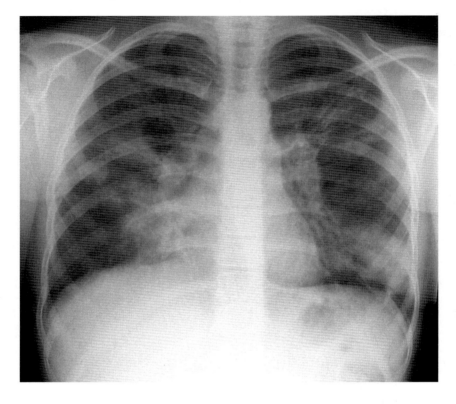

6.2   What is the most likely diagnosis?

- [ ] A *Pseudomonas aeruginosa* infection
- [ ] B Viral pneumonitis
- [ ] C Allergic bronchopulmonary aspergillosis
- [ ] D *Burkholderia cepacia* infection
- [ ] E Atypical mycobacterium infection
- [ ] F *Staphylococcus aureus* infection
- [ ] G Tuberculosis
- [ ] H *Haemophilus influenzae* infection
- [ ] I Asthma
- [ ] J Worsening cystic fibrosis per se
- [ ] K *Mycoplasma pneumoniae* infection
- [ ] L Sarcoidosis

6.3   Which THREE of the following tests will confirm the diagnosis?

- [ ] A   Serum IgE
- [ ] B   Exercise test
- [ ] C   Heaf test
- [ ] D   Early morning urine
- [ ] E   Gastric aspirate
- [ ] F   Radioallergosorbent test to *Aspergillus*
- [ ] G   Sputum culture for *Burkholderia cepacia*
- [ ] H   Paired serum samples for viral titres
- [ ] I   Sputum viral culture
- [ ] J   Lung biopsy
- [ ] K   High resolution CT scan lung
- [ ] L   Serum IgM
- [ ] M   Histamine challenge test
- [ ] N   Serum angiotensin converting enzyme (ACE)
- [ ] O   Sputum culture for *Mycobacteria*
- [ ] P   Nasopharyngeal aspirate
- [ ] Q   Aspergillus precipitins
- [ ] R   Bronchoalveolar lavage

6.4   Which ONE of the following options would you recommend next?

- [ ] A   Oral steroid
- [ ] B   Oral ciprofloxacin
- [ ] C   Intravenous ciprofloxacin and an aminoglycoside
- [ ] D   Oral flucloxacillin
- [ ] E   Intravenous flucloxacillin
- [ ] F   Oral ciprofloxacin and a macrolide
- [ ] G   Inhaled steroid with B$_2$ agonist prn
- [ ] H   Triple antituberculous treatment
- [ ] I   Oral Augmentin
- [ ] J   Careful observation at home – no specific treatment as yet
- [ ] K   Intravenous meropenem and an aminoglycoside

Answers to Question 6 are on page 54

ANSWERS TO QUESTION 6

6.1 F She has a degree of small airways obstruction
    G Her lung function is worse now compared with 1 year ago
    H She has a mixed obstructive-restrictive picture
6.2 C Allergic bronchopulmonary aspergillosis
6.3 A Serum IgE
    F Radioallergosorbent test to *Aspergillus*
    Q Aspergillus precipitins
6.4 A Oral steroid

Discussion

Children with cystic fibrosis often have low-grade persistent pulmonary inflammation that worsens in association with increased numbers of bacteria in airway secretions or as a result of viral infection. This is usually accompanied by increased cough and sputum production (with a change in sputum colour), reduced exercise tolerance, lethargy, anorexia and sometimes a reduction in lung function. Associated fever is unusual and chest examination findings may not have deviated from baseline. Classic teaching describes an escalation of infection from normal respiratory pathogens in the relatively normal lung to progressively more opportunistic pathogens as the CF lung becomes more damaged with time (*Streptococcus pneumoniae, Haemophilus influenzae, Staphylococcus aureus, Pseudomonas aeruginosa, Burkholderia cepacia*). In reality, simultaneous infection with more than one organism may well occur. *S. aureus* and streptococcal species are among the commonest bacteria responsible. Infection with pseudomonas species may occur at any age and typically results in a decline in lung function, which may be irreversible if prompt treatment is not initiated. The mainstays of treatment comprise intensive physiotherapy (at least twice per day) accompanied by a minimum of 2 weeks of antibiotic therapy. A cough swab or sputum culture should be obtained to facilitate an appropriate choice of antibiotic. Previous cough swab/sputum cultures should serve as guide to therapy. If the increase in cough is of short duration (a few days) and the child is otherwise well, oral antibiotic(s) are appropriate. Treatment for *Pseudomonas aeruginosa* (oral ciprofloxacin) should be given to any child known to have previously grown the organism, and nebulised colomycin is a useful adjunct in those children who are not already receiving it.

Failure to improve with intensive physiotherapy and oral antibiotic treatment should prompt an urgent clinical review. If the exacerbation fails to settle after 3 weeks of antibiotics, or has occurred on a background of general deterioration (often including weight loss), a course of intravenous antibiotics may be warranted. Dual therapy with two antipseudomonal antibiotics (eg ceftazidime and gentamicin) is usual practice, though the precise choice of agents is dictated by past and present cough swab culture results. Failure to respond in this case should prompt consideration of an alternative aetiology.

Allergic bronchopulmonary aspergillosis (ABPA) is the consequence of an abnormal immune response to infection with *Aspergillus fumigatus*, and affects up to 10% of children with CF, peaking in teenage years. It may present with an acute deterioration unresponsive to antibiotics or insidiously with no obvious symptoms. Failure to treat it effectively may result in worsening bronchiectasis. Confirming the diagnosis may be difficult. Some CF centres screen for ABPA annually by assessing: history of wheeze, CXR changes, presence of precipitins to aspergillus (IgG), IgE-specific aspergillus (radioallergosorbent test, RAST), total IgE (> 500 IU/litre) and eosinophil count (> 500/µl). The presence of aspergillus in the sputum is not discriminatory, and the number of criteria required to make a diagnosis remains contentious.

Treatment usually comprises non-enteric-coated prednisolone for at least 2 weeks. Once a response is evident (clinical improvement, reduction in IgE of > 35%), the dose can be reduced. Itraconazole is useful in those that fail to respond.

Tuberculous or atypical mycobacterial infection should also be considered in a child with cystic fibrosis with worsening chest symptoms, and can sometimes be confirmed by specific sputum culture and placement of a Heaf/Mantoux test. Antibiotic therapy should be directed by the results of initial investigation and later by culture sensitivity testing.

QUESTION 7

You review a 13-month-old boy in clinic who has been followed up since birth for failure to thrive. He was born at term by normal delivery with no perinatal complications except prolonged jaundice, which finally resolved at 10 weeks of age. A prolonged jaundice screen was unremarkable. Over the first year of life, he has had persistent problems with severe constipation, poor feeding and irritability. He was seen in cardiology clinic at 6 months of age with an asymptomatic murmur diagnosed as trivial pulmonary stenosis. Weight, length and head circumference have been below and parallel to the 0.4th centile.

From a developmental perspective he rolled at 7 months, sat unsupported at 9 months, and sat unaided from 10 months. He is not yet pulling to stand or crawling and is unkeen to weight bear. He started picking up objects at 6 months of age and manipulating two objects at once at 10 months. He cannot hold two objects in one hand. He has a radial approach tripod pincer grip bilaterally but is unable to hold a spoon effectively. He is not casting but is beginning to release objects deliberately. There are no concerns regarding his hearing or vision; he has polysyllabic babble and understands 'no'. He first smiled at 9 weeks, is an affectionate child with his mother and waves bye-bye. He has grasped the concept of object permanence.

On examination he has lost weight (see below). He has a grade 3/6 long systolic murmur radiating from the suprasternal region to his back and right axilla. He has truncal hypotonia and joint laxity. He has palpable stool in the left iliac fossa. Anal margin looks normal. Physical examination is otherwise unremarkable.

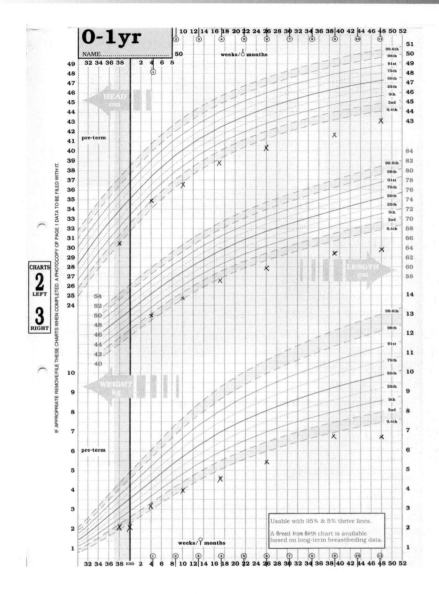

7.1 Estimate his global developmental age

- [ ] A   3–6 months
- [ ] B   6–9 months
- [ ] C   9–12 months
- [ ] D   12–15 months
- [ ] E   15 months+

7.2 Which modality is he most delayed in?

☐ A Gross motor
☐ B Fine motor and vision
☐ C Hearing and speech
☐ D Social/personal development

7.3 Which TEN of the following first-line investigations would you request?

☐ A Full blood count
☐ B Renal function tests
☐ C Liver function tests
☐ D Parathyroid hormone
☐ E Calcium biochemistry
☐ F Sweat test
☐ G Glucose tolerance test
☐ H Thyroid function tests
☐ I Karyotype
☐ J Serum ammonia
☐ K Beta-oxybutyrate
☐ L Urinary amino acids and organic acids
☐ M Early morning cortisol
☐ N Caeruloplasmin
☐ O Serum copper
☐ P Creatine kinase
☐ Q Galactose-1-phosphate uridyl transferase (GAL-1-PUT)
☐ R CT brain
☐ S EEG
☐ T Chest X-ray
☐ U Abdominal X-ray
☐ V Barium enema
☐ W Skin biopsy
☐ X Liver biopsy

Blood results reveal a urea of 8.8 and creatinine 40. A renal ultrasound is requested which reveals bilateral nephrocalcinosis.

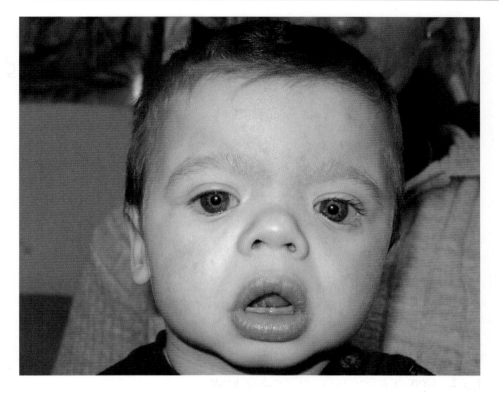

Aged 18 months

7.4   What is the underlying diagnosis?

. . . .

7.5   How would you confirm this diagnosis?

. . . .

ANSWERS TO QUESTION 7

7.1 C 9–12 months
7.2 A Gross motor
7.3 A Full blood count
    B Renal function tests
    C Liver function tests
    E Calcium biochemistry
    F Sweat test
    H Thyroid function tests
    I Karyotype
    L Urinary amino acids and organic acids
    P Creatine kinase
    U Abdominal X-ray
7.4 Williams' syndrome
7.5 Fluorescent in-situ hybridisation (FISH) for Williams' syndrome

Discussion

Developmental milestones are conveniently divided into four modalities – gross motor, fine motor and vision, hearing and speech, personal/social development.
    Milestones mentioned in this case:

Milestones	Age
Gross motor milestones	
Rolling	5–7 months
Sitting	from 6 months
Sitting unaided	7–8 months
Pulling to stand	9 months
Crawling	9–11 months
Fine motor milestones	
Palmar grasp	6 months
Transferring objects	7–8 months
Intermediate (tripod) grasp	9 months
Controlled release of object	10 months
Mature pincer grip	10–12 months

| Casting | 12 months |
| Two objects in one hand | 13 months |

Hearing and speech

| Polysyllabic babble | 10–12 months |
| Understands 'no' | 10–12 months |

Social/personal

Shows affection	10–12 months
Waves bye-bye	10–12 months
Object permanence	9–12 months

This boy has a gross motor developmental profile of 8 months, fine motor profile at 9–10 months, language at 11–12 months and social development at about 12 months.

Williams' syndrome is a sporadic congenital syndrome caused by a microdeletion of chromosome 7 at the elastin gene locus. Incidence is 1:20,000. It is a multisystem disorder, the principal components of which are:

Idiopathic infantile hypercalcaemia
- Hypercalcaemia/hypercalciuria present in 70%
- Normalises by 18 months; may recur in puberty
- May cause metastatic calcification (kidney, bones)

Cardiovascular disease
- Supravalvar aortic stenosis   50%
- Peripheral pulmonary stenosis   20%
- VSD   10%

Mild to severe learning difficulties   97%
- IQ 55–70; ability in reading, writing and arithmetic tends to peak age 8–10 years

Classic elfin-like facies – broad forehead, full cheeks and lips, prominent philtrum, wide mouth, peg teeth, flat nasal bridge, hypertelorism and stellate iris

Distinct behavioural phenotype – language attainment is initially slow; however, enhanced mimicry skills and social interest give people with Williams' syndrome precocious, highly social, fluent but superficial language – the 'cocktail personality'

Irritability, poor feeding, failure to thrive and profound constipation with or without rectal prolapse are common in the first year of life. The diagnosis can easily be overlooked in this age group, as the classic facial appearance tends to develop after 2 years of age, becoming more pronounced with time.

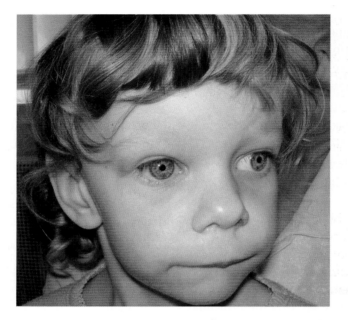

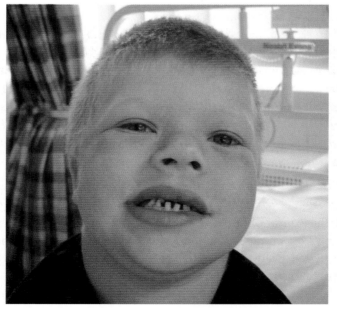

QUESTION 8

Consider the following disorders

A   Partial AVSD

B   Transposition of the great arteries with intact ventricular septum and a restrictive foramen ovale

C   Tetralogy of Fallot

D   Truncus arteriosus

E   Obstructed total anomalous pulmonary venous drainage

F   Persistent fetal circulation

G   Pulmonary atresia/stenosis

H   Ebstein's anomaly

I   Tricuspid atresia

J   Hypoplastic left heart syndrome

K   AVSD

L   VSD with high pulmonary vascular resistance

M   Ostium secundum ASD

N   Coarctation of the aorta

O   Cor triatriatum

P   Aortic stenosis

Case I

You are called urgently to the delivery suite to review a baby boy who is 8 minutes old and has already been intubated. He is now being hand-bagged on the resuscitaire. He was born by forceps delivery at 38 weeks gestation after labour had failed to progress and vacuum extraction had been unsuccessful. CTG immediately prior to delivery showed some late decelerations. There was some light meconium-staining of the liquor but none evident on subglottic aspiration. He had cried briefly at birth but remained blue despite facial oxygen and then mask ventilation, and so was intubated at 4 minutes of age by the attending doctor.

His mother is an insulin-dependent diabetic whose control has been generally good this pregnancy. Booking serology was unremarkable and the anomaly scan was normal at 21 weeks. Serial growth scans in the 2nd and 3rd trimesters were normal. Membranes ruptured 4 hours prior to delivery and her highest temperature in labour was 37.7°C. She has never had a high vaginal swab. There is no family history of note. Mother's first child is a fit and well 3-year-old girl.

On examination he looks cyanosed. He is being hand-ventilated while you examine him but when he is disconnected from the bag, his respiratory rate is approximately 55. Air entry is adequate and breath sounds are normal. Pulse oximetry saturation on his right hand is 82% in 10 litres of oxygen/minute. All peripheral pulses are palpable. Heart rate is 160. He has a systolic murmur audible along the left sternal border. Perfusion is good. His liver is palpable 1 cm below the right mid-costal margin. Tone is intermittently increased and he is generally active. You elect to transfer him to the neonatal unit and on admission he is given a 0.4 mg morphine bolus and started on synchronised intermittent mandatory ventilation (SIMV). Initial settings are: pressure 18/4, rate 30, inspiratory time 0.4, FiO$_2$ 0.6. Mean arterial blood pressure is 39 mmHg (right arm), 41 mmHg (left leg). He is apyrexial.

His right radial artery is cannulated and an arterial blood gas obtained (pH 7.38, pCO$_2$ 3.9 kPa, pO$_2$ 4.0 kPa, HCO$_3^-$ 21, base excess −4). Despite increasing ventilatory support he remains cyanosed. A chest X-ray is taken. He does not receive surfactant therapy.

8.1 Which of the following descriptions best describes the SIMV mode of ventilation?

☐ A He receives a minimum of 30 breaths per minute, each of a peak pressure of 18 cm H$_2$O and each 0.4 s long. If he initiates a breath 30 times in a minute, he only receives 30 breaths. If he initiates more than one breath every 2 s, each additional breath during a 2-s period is also supported with a peak pressure of 18 cm H$_2$O and is 0.4 s long.

☐ B He receives a minimum of 30 breaths per minute, each of a peak pressure of 18 cm H$_2$O and each 0.4 s long. If he initiates a breath 30 times in a minute, he receives only 30 breaths, each breath is pressure-generated and the pressure is delivered when he initiates a breath. If he initiates more than one breath in a 2-s period, any additional breath is not pressure-supported and the tidal volume generated is dependent on his own respiratory effort.

☐ C He receives 30 breaths per minute, pressure-generated to a peak of 18 cm H$_2$O, each 0.4 s long, each every 2 s. Any breath he takes is not pressure-supported and the tidal volume generated is dependent on his own respiratory effort.

☐ D He receives a minimum of 30 breaths per minute, each of a peak pressure of 18 cm H$_2$O and each 0.4 s long. If he initiates a breath 30 times in a minute, he receives only 30 breaths, though each breath is pressure-generated by the ventilator. If he initiates more than one breath in a 2-s period, any additional breath is supported by the ventilator with a peak pressure of 18 cm H_2O, but the I-time for each of these additional breaths is self-generated and the tidal volume variable.

☐ E He receives a continuous positive end expiratory pressure (PEEP) of 4 cm H_2O. Each breath he takes is supported by the ventilator with a peak pressure of 18 cm H_2O. The I-time for each of his breaths is not fixed. His tidal volume varies with each breath, as does his minute volume.

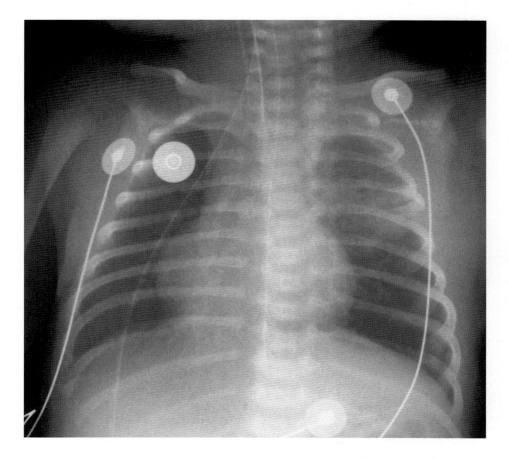

Chest X-ray

In view of his cyanosis an ECG is requested.

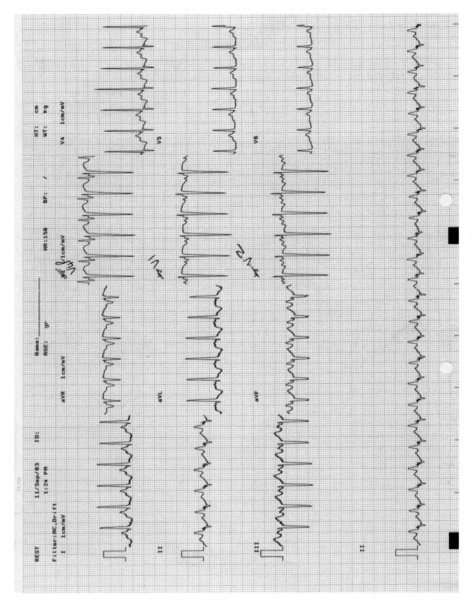

ECG

8.2   Within which range does the mean frontal axis lie?

A   0 to 60°
B   −60° to 120°
C   60° to 120°
D   120° to 180°
E   0° to −60°
F   −120° to −180°

A nitrogen washout test is undertaken. The results are as follows:

	Right radial artery	Umbilical artery catheter
Pre washout test		
pH	7.34	7.32
pCO_2	3.5 kPa	3.7 kPa
pO_2	3.6 kPa	3.9 kPa
HCO_3^-	20	21
Base excess	−5	−4
Post washout test		
pH	7.34	7.32
pCO_2	3.9 kPa	3.7 kPa
pO_2	3.9 kPa	3.9 kPa
HCO_3^-	21	20
Base excess	−4	−5

8.3   Select the most likely diagnosis for this child from the list of disorders on p. 63

. . . .

Case 2

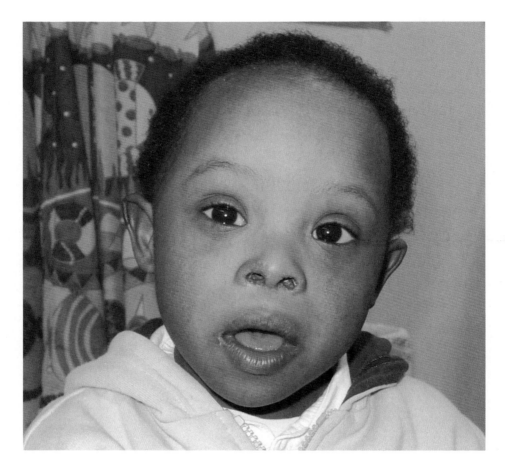

History: Symptom-free

Examination: Pink, normal pulses, right arm blood pressure 80/50, fixed splitting of S_2, systolic murmur at base of the heart, chest clear

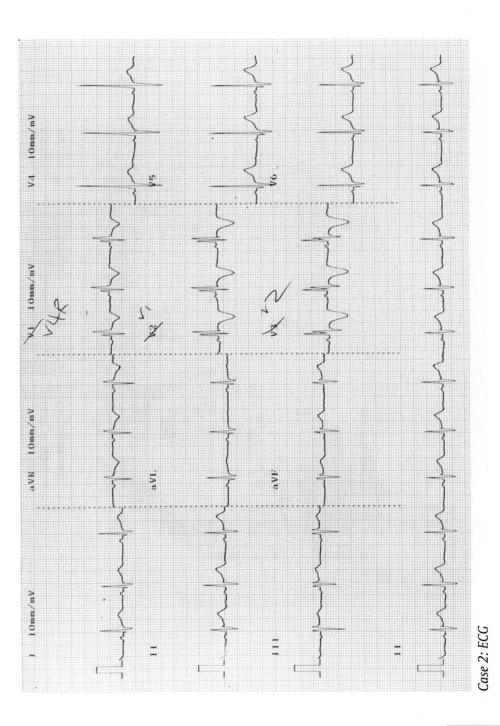

Case 2: ECG

8.4 From the list of disorders on p. 63, select the most likely one for the child illustrated on p. 68.

. . . .

Case 3

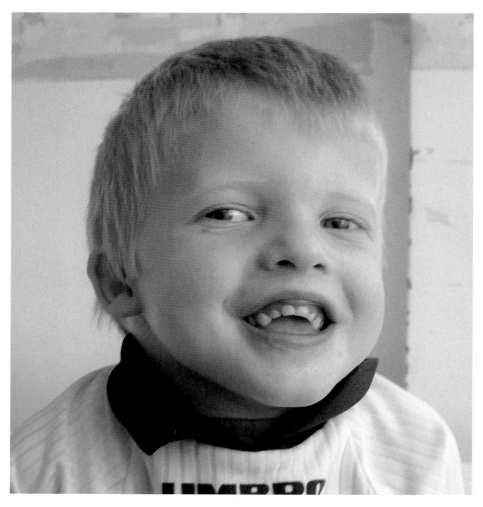

History: Mild cyanosis and murmur noted at 6-week check. Surgery at 3 months (palliative) and then at 9 months (corrective). Now symptom-free

Examination: Pink. Normal pulses. Systolic and diastolic murmur over upper left sternal edge. RR20. No hepatomegaly

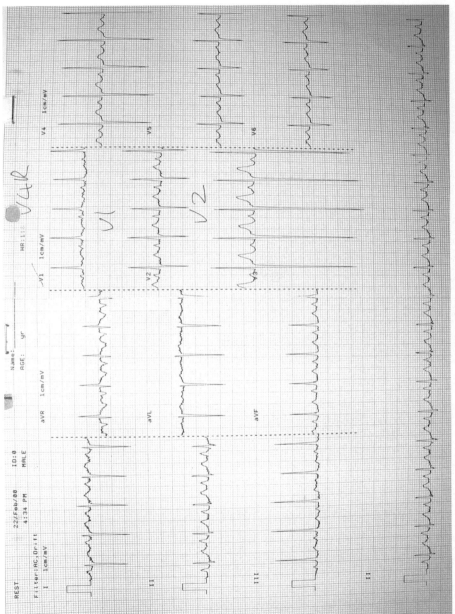

Case 3: ECG

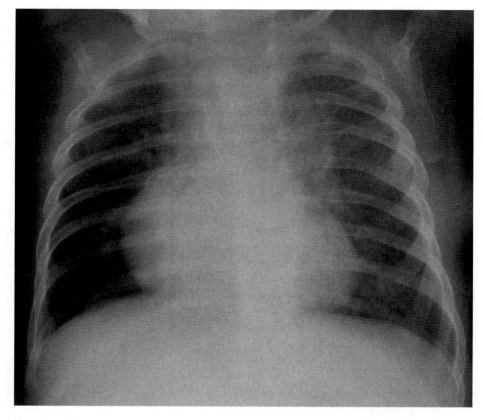

Case 3: CXR

8.5 Select the most likely diagnosis for this child from the list of disorders on p. 63

. . . .

8.6 Suggest a possible underlying diagnosis.

. . . .

Case 4

8.7 Select the most likely diagnosis for this child from the list of disorders on p. 63

History: 1-day-old term baby noted to be blue on 1st day check

Examination: Oxygen saturations 62% in air. Normal four-limb pulses. Blood pressure 45/32. No murmur. RR 70. Breath sounds vesicular Liver 1 cm. When started on intravenous prostaglandin he becomes more tachypnoeic without improvement in oxygen saturation. Venous pH 7.26, pCO_2 6.2 kPa, pO_2 2.2 kPa, HCO_3^- 20, base excess −5

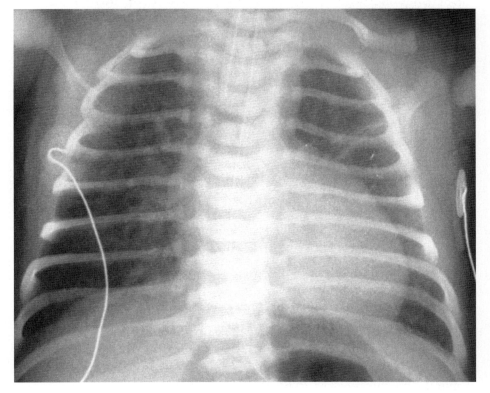

Chest x-ray

Answers to Question 8 are on page 74

ANSWERS TO QUESTION 8

Case 1

8.1 B   He receives a minimum of 30 breaths per minute, each of a peak pressure of 18 cm H_2O and each 0.4 s long. If he initiates a breath 30 times in a minute, he receives only 30 breaths, each breath is pressure-generated and the pressure is delivered when he initiates a breath. If he initiates more than one breath in a 2-s period, any additional breath is not pressure-supported and the tidal volume generated is dependent on his own respiratory effort.

8.2 E   0° to –60°

8.3 I   Tricuspid atresia

Case 2

8.4 A   Ostium primum ASD

Case 3

8.5 C   Tetralogy of Fallot

8.6   DiGeorge syndrome

Case 4

8.7 B   Transposition of the great arteries with intact ventricular septum and a restrictive foramen ovale

Discussion

Case 1

The ventilatory modes outlined in Question 8.1 are as follows:

A Synchronised intermittent positive pressure (SIPPV)
He receives a minimum of 30 breaths per minute, each of a peak pressure of 18 cm H_2O and each 0.4 s long. If he initiates a breath 30 times in a minute, he only receives 30 breaths. If he initiates more than one breath every 2 s, each additional breath during a 2-s period is also supported with a peak pressure of 18 cm H_2O and is 0.4 s long.

B Synchronised intermittent mandatory ventilation (SIMV)
He receives a minimum of 30 breaths per minute, each of a peak pressure of 18 cm H_2O and each 0.4 s long. If he initiates a breath 30 times in a minute, he receives only 30 breaths, each breath is pressure-generated

and the pressure is delivered when he initiates a breath. If he initiates more than one breath in a 2-s period, any additional breath is not pressure-supported and the tidal volume generated is dependent on his own respiratory effort.

C Continuous mandatory ventilation (CMV)

He receives 30 breaths per minute, pressure-generated to a peak of 18 cm H_2O, each 0.4 s long, each every 2 s. Any breath he takes is not pressure-supported and the tidal volume generated is dependent on his own respiratory effort.

D SIMV + pressure support/ASB

He receives a minimum of 30 breaths per minute, each of a peak pressure of 18 cm H_2O and each 0.4 s long. If he initiates a breath 30 times in a minute, he receives only 30 breaths, though each breath is pressure-generated by the ventilator. If he initiates more than one breath in a 2-s period, any additional breath is supported by the ventilator with a peak pressure of 18 cm H_2O, but the I-time for each of these additional breaths is self-generated and the tidal volume variable.

E CPAP with ASB

He receives a continuous positive end expiratory pressure of (PEEP) of 4 cmH_2O. Each breath he takes is supported by the ventilator with a peak pressure of 18 cm H_2O. The I-time for each of his breaths is not fixed. His tidal volume varies with each breath, as does his minute volume.

From the history provided this baby may have been at risk for hypoxic ischaemic encephalopathy following birth. The CTG showed late decelerations, there was some meconium-staining of the liquor and mother required a forceps-assisted delivery. However, this baby cried at birth and is active on the resuscitaire once intubated, which mediates against severe in-utero hypoxia and greatly reduces the likelihood of persistent fetal circulation.

The history suggests he was intubated because of cyanosis rather than respiratory distress or apnoea. There are no risk factors for neonatal infection (term gestation, no prolonged rupture of membranes, no maternal fever, no neonatal infection in a previous pregnancy and no documented Group B streptococcus birth tract colonisation). The most important clinical findings are the marked cyanosis refractory to oxygen therapy, and a murmur, which together suggest congenital cyanotic heart disease. The six major causes of congenital cyanotic heart disease which present early in the neonatal period are:

- Pulmonary atresia or critical pulmonary stenosis
- Transposition of the great arteries (TGA with an intact ventricular septum is usually 'murmurless')
- Ebstein's anomaly
- Severe Tetralogy of Fallot (although severe cyanosis is unusual in early life)
- Obstructed total anomalous pulmonary venous drainage
- Tricuspid atresia

It is also important to exclude primary respiratory disease although the gestation, history, initial blood gas and chest X-ray collectively mediate against this. Finally, methaemoglobinaemia should not be forgotten but is an extremely rare cause of perceived 'cyanosis', and there are other far more likely diagnoses in this baby. Careful examination of the ECG seals the diagnosis, as the presence of a leftward axis, right atrial hypertrophy and an absence of right ventricular forces is pathognomonic of tricuspid atresia in this clinical context.

If echocardiography is not readily available a hyperoxia (nitrogen washout) test can be carried out on neonates with visible cyanosis, circulatory collapse or a resting pulse oximetry reading of < 95%. A baseline right radial (preductal) arterial blood gas is first obtained with the baby breathing air, and then repeated with the child inspiring 100% oxygen. Pulse oximetry should be documented at preductal and postductal sites to assess for reverse or differential cyanosis. In some neonates with severe pulmonary disease, the hyperoxia test must be performed using positive pressure ventilation as they may not be able to raise their PaO_2 unless ventilated. Pulse oximetry should **not** be used for interpretation of the hyperoxia test because the results can be dangerously misleading. The test can be interpreted as follows:

	FiO$_2$ = 0.21 PaO$_2$ kPa (% saturation)		FiO$_2$ = 1.00 PaO$_2$ kPa (% saturation)	PaCO$_2$ kPa
Normal	10 (95)		>40 (100)	5
Pulmonary disease	7 (85)		>20 (100)	7
Methaemoglobinaemia	10 (95)		>25 (100)	5
Cardiac disease				
Parallel circulation[1]	<5 (<75)		<6.5 (<85)	5
Mixing with restricted pulmonary				
blood flow[2]	<5 (<75)		<6.5 (<85)	5
Mixing without restricted				
pulmonary blood flow[3]	6.5–8 (85–93)		<20 (<100)	5
	Preductal	*Postductal*		
Differential cyanosis[4]	10 (95)	5 (<75)	Variable	5–7
Reverse differential Cyanosis	<5 (<75)	10 (95)	Variable	5–7

[1] TGA with/without intact ventricular septum ✔
[2] Tricuspid atresia with pulmonary stenosis or atresia, critical pulmonary stenosis or pulmonary atresia with intact ventricular septum, Tetralogy of Fallot
[3] Truncus arteriosûs, TAPVD, hypoplastic left heart syndrome, single ventricle
[4] Left ventricular outflow tract obstruction, persistent pulmonary hypertension of the newborn
[5] TGA with coarctation of the aorta or interrupted aortic arch, TGA with pulmonary hypertension

(Adapted from Barone, M.A. (ed.) 1996. *The Harriet Lane Handbook*, 14th edn. St Louis, Mosby, p.155.)

Congenital cyanotic heart disease presenting early in life is likely be duct-dependant. An intravenous infusion of prostaglandin E1 or E2 should be started and the opinion of a paediatric cardiologist sought at the first opportunity.

Case 2

This child has Down's syndrome. 40% of children with this condition will have congenital heart disease. Of these, 43% will typically have a complete AVSD, 32% a VSD, 10% an ASD, 6% tetralogy of Fallot, 4% isolated persistent patency of the arterial duct and 5% other lesions. (This ECG shows right bundle branch block (rSR in V$_1$) with left axis deviation, and these findings together with the fixed split second heart sound and a murmur make a partial AVSD the most likely diagnosis) *

Case 3

This child has DiGeorge syndrome. Tetralogy of Fallot is a well-recognised association in children with this condition and is supported in this case by the history and the evidence of right ventricular hypertrophy both on ECG (everted 'T' waves in V$_1$ and V$_2$) and chest X-ray. *

Case 4

In a blue baby with no murmur, and an egg-shaped heart with a narrow
mediastinum on chest X-ray, the most likely diagnosis is TGA with intact
ventricular septum.)The position of the aorta lying behind the pulmonary
artery is responsible for this X-ray appearance. In this situation, mixing occurs
at the level of the PDA and at atrial level through the foramen ovale. Flow at
ductal level is mostly from aorta to pulmonary artery as pressures in the aorta
are higher than in the pulmonary artery. This increases flow in the pulmonary
circulation and back to the left side of the heart as a consequence. Babies
with this condition who also have a restrictive foramen ovale may become
more breathless when a prostaglandin infusion is started, as the left atrium
becomes overloaded, increasing pulmonary venous pressure.

QUESTION 9

An 11-year-old boy is referred to the neurology outpatient clinic because his parents are worried he has developed epilepsy. Over the last 2 months he has been complaining that his tongue and gums have occasionally been feeling 'funny' in the morning. During one such episode he also experienced contractions of his lower face and jerking of his left hand. He did not fall to the floor or lose consciousness, was not incontinent and has a good recollection of this episode. Two further episodes have apparently occurred at night, witnessed by his older brother with whom he shares a bedroom.

He is otherwise fit and well. He denies headaches, vomiting, visual disturbance or focal weakness. He has not lost weight. He is on no medication. He was born at term and spent one day in the special care baby unit because he was slow to feed after birth. He has recently started in a mainstream school where he has unfortunately been bullied. Family history is unremarkable except that his father developed generalised epilepsy in his twenties.

Physical examination is unremarkable.

EEG

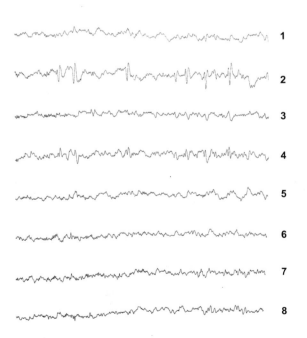

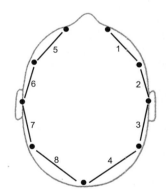

9.1 What is the most likely diagnosis?

- [ ] A Pseudoseizures
- [ ] B Idiopathic generalised epilepsy
- [ ] C BECTS (benign epilepsy with centrotemporal spikes)
- [ ] D Autosomal dominant nocturnal frontal epilepsy
- [ ] E Night terrors
- [ ] F CNS malignancy
- [ ] G Complex partial seizures
- [ ] H Myoclonic epilepsy
- [ ] I Landau–Kleffner syndrome
- [ ] J Temporal lobe epilepsy

9.2 Which ONE of the following is the most appropriate next step in management?

- [ ] A No treatment, review again in outpatients
- [ ] B Carbamazepine
- [ ] C Phenobarbitone
- [ ] D CT scan brain
- [ ] E Admit for continuous telemetry
- [ ] F Ethosuximide
- [ ] E Sodium valproate
- [ ] F Vigabatrin
- [ ] G Psychology referral

Answers to Question 9 are on page 82

ANSWERS TO QUESTION 9

9.1 C BECTS (Benign epilepsy with centrotemporal spikes)
9.2 A No treatment, review again in outpatients

Discussion

The history and EEG findings are absolutely typical of BECTS (benign epilepsy with centrotemporal spikes). This condition was previously known as benign rolandic epilepsy, a common type of partial epilepsy with an excellent prognosis. It typically occurs in otherwise normal children between the ages of 2 and 14 years, with a peak age of onset of 9–10 years. Seizures occur during sleep or on awakening. As in this case, the seizures are usually partial but secondary generalisation may occur especially during sleep.

Somatosensory symptoms and motor signs are usually confined to the face. Unilateral paraesthesia is followed by tonic and/or clonic contractions of the tongue, lips, cheek, larynx and pharynx, and sometimes the ipsilateral upper extremity. Dysphagia is a common complaint. Most children have infrequent seizures, and in 75% of cases seizures occur only in sleep (An anticonvulsant (carbamazepine is the preferred agent) is reserved for those in whom daytime seizures are problematic or in those children experiencing significant sleep disturbance as a result of seizures. Seizures usually cease spontaneously by puberty.) *

In this question, none of the other differential diagnoses are likely. His seizures are not generalised or myoclonic. Complex partial seizures are accompanied by impaired consciousness, which is not a feature in this case. Temporal lobe epilepsy is synonymous with complex partial seizures. Autosomal dominant nocturnal frontal epilepsy manifests as night-time seizures associated with sleep disturbance (bad dreams, feelings of sudden fear, self-perception of difficulty in breathing) usually with a positive family history of parasomnia or somnambulism. A lack of symptoms suggestive of intracranial pathology (headaches, vomiting, visual disturbance, focal weakness), coupled with a normal physical examination do not support a diagnosis of CNS malignancy. Landau–Kleffner syndrome is characterised by regression of language skills around 5 years of age in a previously normal child, quite unlike the case presented.

QUESTION 10

As the paediatric registrar on call, you are asked to review a 7-month-old child who has been brought by his grandmother to the A&E department for assessment. Whilst looking after him she has become concerned about the shape of his right leg. She has been looking after him all that afternoon whilst his mother and father have gone to work.

His grandmother says that she has not noticed his bent leg before, and isn't sure whether it was like that when his mother dropped him off earlier that afternoon. She has contacted the mother by phone and she herself is now en-route to the hospital to find out what has been going on. His grandmother says that whilst in her care he has been happy and smiling and has taken one 6 oz bottle of formula milk uneventfully. He has only been out of her sight once, when she went to the toilet leaving him strapped in a custom-made baby chair for about 5 minutes. There have been no visitors to the house that afternoon, and grandfather has been out since 2 pm. She noticed his bent leg when she changed his nappy after feeding him.

As you are continuing your assessment, the infant's mother arrives in the department and is clearly very cross with grandmother, although it is not entirely clear why at that point. You are able to ascertain from mother that he was a breech presentation, born at 36 weeks gestation by emergency caesarean section after unsuccessful cephalic version. He required a brief spell in facial oxygen at birth but was not admitted to NICU and was discharged home on day 2 after a normal first day check. Birth weight was 3.1 kg (50th centile), head circumference 35 cm (90th centile). Early infancy had proceeded unremarkably until about 5 days ago when his mother thinks she first noticed his 'funny leg'. She was planning to ask her health visitor about it when she next visited the family centre later this week. She has five other children aged 11, 9, 6, 4 and 2 years of age. The 11-year-old child has been statemented but attends mainstream school. Father has high blood pressure and is on some tablets but apparently has no other medical problems. There is no other family history of note.

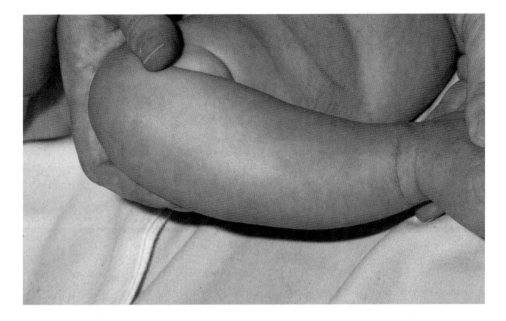

On examination he is not dysmorphic. Weight is 7.5 kg (25–50th centile), head circumference 47.9 cm (just above 98th centile). Fontanelle is soft. Pulse is 110 beats per minute, blood pressure 60/40, heart sounds are normal with no murmurs. Respiratory examination is normal. He has 1.5 cm hepatomegaly but no splenomegaly. You find his developmental examination to be just about concordant with that of a 6-month-old infant.

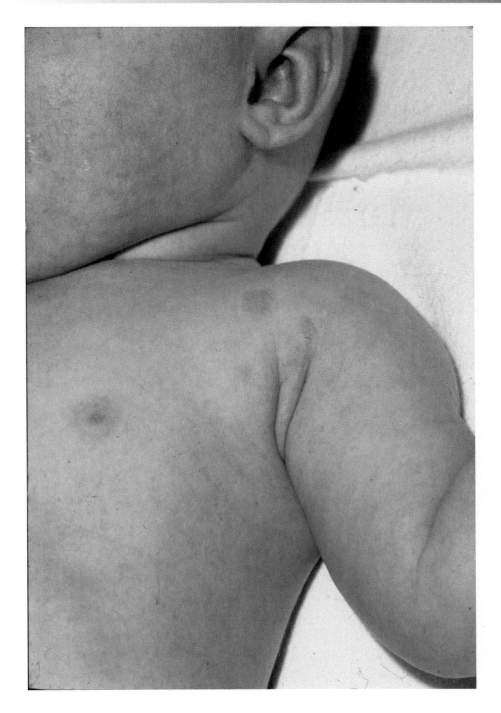

10.1 **With the results of his developmental examination in mind, which five of the following is he most likely to be able to do?**

☐ A   Sit without support
☐ B   Roll from stomach to back
☐ C   Transfer objects
☐ D   Turn towards a voice
☐ E   Say 'dada'
☐ F   Smile at a mirror
☐ G   Frolic when played with
☐ H   Ring a bell
☐ I   Throw an object
☐ J   Make consonant sounds
☐ K   Search for lost objects

You request an X-ray of his right leg. This film is reviewed by the on-call orthopaedic registrar who reports it as showing a healed fracture of the tibia and fibula. It is now 7 pm.

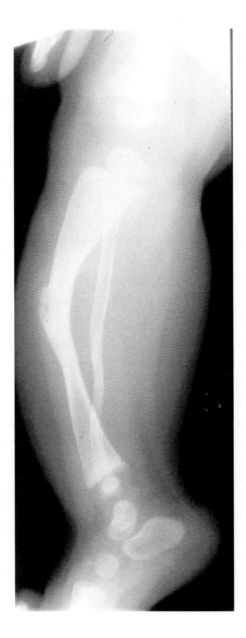

10.2 With this in mind, after notifying the consultant paediatrician on call, what would be the next most appropriate management step?

☐ A Refer on to the named consultant for child protection at your trust, on suspicion of non-accidental injury

☐ B Refer to social services for an opinion, on suspicion of non-accidental injury

☐ C Seek a formal radiological opinion before embarking on further management

☐ D Carry out a metabolic bone screen

☐ E Refer directly to the local Police Child Protection team

☐ F Discharge home overnight, but arrange to review again on the ward tomorrow

☐ G Request a skeletal survey

☐ H Request that the on-call orthopaedic team take over this child's care

10.3 In light of the leg examination and X-ray, what would be the next most appropriate step in management with regard to this child's head circumference?

☐ A Cranial USS to exclude chronic subdural haematomas

☐ B CT scan to exclude chronic subdural haematomas

☐ C Examine the parents

☐ D MRI scan to exclude chronic subdural haematomas

☐ E Request ophthalmology opinion with view to retinoscopy

☐ F Skeletal survey

☐ G Refer to a neurosurgeon for an opinion

☐ H No specific attention is required

10.4 Suggest a unifying diagnosis

. . . .

Answers to Question 10 are on page 90

ANSWERS TO QUESTION 10

10.1 B Roll from stomach to back
     C Transfer objects
     D Turn towards a voice
     F Smile at a mirror
     G Frolic when played with
10.2 C Seek a formal radiological opinion before embarking on further management
10.3 C Examine the parents
10.4   Neurofibromatosis type I (NF-I)

Discussion

This question illustrates the importance of obtaining an expert opinion on any investigation performed in a child in whom the diagnosis of non-accidental injury is being considered. This is a real case in which the right leg was initially considered to be fractured. In the absence of an explanatory history from the child's parents, a referral to the child protection team was made on the night of admission. This was retracted the following morning when a paediatric radiologist noted that the X-ray demonstrated abnormal bone, compatible with that seen in NF-I, which in this case had precipitated the formation of a pseudoarthrosis.

*   There are other clues in this history and examination that might prompt consideration of NF-I. Relative macrocephaly with a soft fontanelle, café-au-lait patches on the trunk and leg, and a family history of macrocephaly with hypertension in father also supports the diagnosis.

Diagnostic criteria for neurofibromatosis type I

Two of the following:

- six or more café-au-lait spots over 5 mm in diameter in prepubertal children and over 15 mm in postpubertal children
- axillary or inguinal freckling
- two or more Lisch nodules on the iris
- two or more neurofibromas or one plexiform neurofibroma
- a distinctive osseous lesion, eg. cortical thinning of long bones with or without pseudoarthrosis; scoliosis
- optic glioma(s)

In the outpatient setting regular assessment of growth parameters, eyes and vision, blood pressure and the musculoskeletal system are mandatory. Macrocephaly in these children may just reflect a large brain, but may also develop secondary to intracranial tumours (usually neurofibromas or astrocytomas) and consequent obstructive hydrocephalus. The diencephalic syndrome occurs as a consequence of a chiasmal glioma compressing the hypothalamus and may cause rapid weight loss. Regular pubertal staging is important as puberty is often precocious or delayed.

Ophthalmic examination may show Lisch nodules (in 90% by age 5 years), optic glioma with consequent proptosis and decreased visual acuity, ptosis from plexiform neuroma of the eyelid and papilloedema secondary to raised intracranial pressure from obstructive hydrocephalus.

Hypertension in NF-I may be due to a number of causes which include coarctation of the aorta, phaeochromocytoma, renal artery stenosis, noradrenaline secreting neurofibromas and essential hypertension.

Skin manifestations are characterized by café-au-lait spots, axillary freckling mid-childhood and the development of multiple peripheral neurofibromas at the onset of puberty.

Of all children presenting with pseudoarthrosis, 60% have NF-I. Conversely only 5% of all children with NF-I will present with pseudoarthrosis. The middle or distal third of the tibia is the commonest site. Scoliosis, pectus excavatum and hemihypertrophy are other common musculoskeletal abnormalities. Long-tract neurological signs may reflect cerebral (eg. tumours), spinal cord (spinal neurofibroma) or peripheral nervous system involvement (eg brachial plexus neurofibromas).

QUESTION 11

Consider the following list of diagnoses – List A

A 21α-hydroxylase deficiency

B 11β-hydroxylase deficiency

C 3β-hydroxysteroid dehydrogenase deficiency

D Complete androgen insensitivity syndrome

E Partial androgen insensitivity syndrome

F 5α-reductase deficiency

G Leydig cell hypoplasia

H Mixed gonadal dysgenesis

I XY pure gonadal dysgenesis

J XX pure gonadal dysgenesis

K Panhypopituitarism

L Kallman's syndrome

M WAGR syndrome

N Denys–Drash syndrome

O Smith–Lemli–Opitz syndrome

Consider the following list of investigations – List B

A Karyotype

B Fluorescent in-situ hybridisation studies

C 17–OH progesterone levels

D Plasma electrolytes

E Pelvic ultrasound

F Adrenal ultrasound

G Cranial ultrasound

H Cystourethrogenitogram

I BHCG test for Dihydrotestosterone/testosterone ratios

J Urinary steroid profile

K Pituitary function tests

L Short synacthen test

M Long synacthen test

N Glucagon stimulation test

Continued on p.93

O   Gonadal biopsy
P   Ophthalmic investigation
Q   LHRH test
R   Testosterone levels
S   Maternal androgens
T   Blood pressure monitoring

Case 1

You are asked to see a 2-day-old child on the postnatal wards with unusual genitalia. Pertinent findings on full examination include a microphallus, bifid scrotum with small palpable testes and normal anus. No female structures are visible on pelvic ultrasound. Karyotype is 46XY. Blood pressure and serum electrolytes are normal. Plasma testosterone levels are elevated.

11.1   From List A, what are the two most likely diagnoses given the above information?

. . . .

. . . .

11.2   From List B, which test will help differentiate the two possible diagnoses?

. . . .

. . . .

Case 2

You are asked to review a 4-day-old child with ambiguous genitalia. The child has a microphallus, fused labioscrotal folds and normal anus. There are no palpable testes. Karyotype is 46XX. Pelvic ultrasound shows normal female structures. Blood pressure 120/80.

11.3   Given the following results, which diagnosis from List A is the most likely?

. . . .

Case 3

You review a 15-year-old girl in clinic with amenorrhoea. Her pubertal staging is B4 P1 A1. Height and weight are on the 25th centile.

11.4 From List A, what is the likely diagnosis?

. . . .

✓Case 4

On first day examination of a term baby, you find ambiguous genitalia and unusually large retinal red reflexes bilaterally. The child has a microphallus, bifid scrotum and normal anus. There are palpable testes.

11.5 From List A what is the likely diagnosis?

. . . .

11.6 Which additional problem should this child be screened for?

. . . .

✓ Case 5

You are called to assess a 5-day-old infant found on the postnatal wards to have a blood glucose of 1.2 mmol/litre. In brief, the child was born at term with no perinatal complications and with a birthweight of 3.1 kg. You resuscitate the child with iv dextrose, iv infusion of fluids and iv antibiotics. On examination the child is found to have a micropenis at 1.5 cm in length, normal scrotum, two palpable testes and normal anus. Examination is otherwise unremarkable with no dysmorphic features. Preliminary investigations show urinary ketones positive, urinary reducing sugars negative; plasma electrolytes reveal hyponatraemia and hyperkalaemia.

11.7 From List A, which is the most likely diagnosis?

. . . .

Case 6

You are asked to see a 3-day-old infant on the postnatal wards with unusual genitalia. Pertinent findings on full examination include a microphallus, bifid scrotum with a single palpable testis and normal anus. There are loose skinfolds at the nape of the neck and pedal oedema. Female structures are visible on pelvic ultrasound. Serum testosterone levels are reduced.

11.8   From List A, what are the most likely diagnoses given the above information?

. . . .

11.9   Which single test from List B will make the diagnosis?

. . . .

Answers to Question 11 are on page 96

ANSWERS TO QUESTION·11

11.1   E, F Partial androgen insensitivity syndrome and 5α-reductase
            deficiency
11.2   I   Beta HCG test for dihydrotestosterone/testosterone ratios
11.3   B   11β-hydroxylase deficiency
11.4   D   Complete androgen insensitivity syndrome
11.5   M   WAGR syndrome
11.6   Wilms' tumour
11.7   K   Panhypopituitarism
11.8   H   Mixed gonadal dysgenesis
11.9   A   Karyotype

Discussion

Case 1

This infant has a male karyotype but is undervirilised. Because testosterone levels are elevated, all conditions relating to defects in testosterone synthesis can be excluded. This includes abnormalities of the hypothalamic–pituitary axis, Leydig cell hypoplasia, and deficiencies in the adrenal/testicular enzyme pathway to testosterone.

(Testosterone is converted to dihydrotestosterone (DHT) by 5α-reductase, and it is DHT which causes virilisation)(In 5α-reductase deficiency, the dihydrotestosterone:testosterone ratio on βHCG stimulation is reduced and virilisation is therefore limited to the weaker direct effect of testosterone. There may be further virilisation at puberty as testosterone levels increase dramatically at this stage.) ✶

The androgen insensitivity syndromes describe a heterogeneous group • of defects in end organ androgen receptor function. Androgen levels are elevated and dihydrotestosterone:testosterone ratio on βHCG stimulation is normal. Partial androgen insensitivity will result in undervirilisation in the male whereas complete androgen insensitivity in the male presents with a female external phenotype (see Case 3).

Case 2

This infant has ambiguous genitalia without palpable testes and is therefore likely to be a virilised female. The most common cause of this presentation is congenital adrenal hyperplasia. This disorder encompasses deficiencies in several enzymes in the adrenal steroid pathway. An enzyme deficiency may have consequences on sex steroid, mineralocorticoid and glucocorticoid production. The commonest cause of virilisation in the female is 21α-hydroxylase deficiency, which blocks production of cortisol and aldosterone. This results in increased levels of ACTH, consequent hypertrophy of the adrenal gland and massive production of the steroid precursor 17-OH progesterone. 17-OH progesterone is shunted down the androgen biosynthesis pathway with consequent virilisation. Deficiency of aldosterone and cortisol means these infants are at risk of addisonian crisis, which in the severe form often presents in the first 10 days of life with hypotension, hypoglycaemia, hyponatraemia and hyperkalaemia. The infant in this case has hypertension in addition to virilised genitalia. 11β-Hydroxylase deficiency is a rare enzyme deficiency in which cortisol production is deficient but the aldosterone pathway is functional. Again there is adrenal hypertrophy and accumulation of intermediates. One of these is deoxycorticosterone (DOC), which is thought to be responsible for the hypertension.

Case 3

Complete androgen insensitivity will result in a female external phenotype. These XY individuals will have produced MIH in utero and consequently female internal genitalia will be absent. These children may present in childhood with a maldescended testis and complete AIS should be suspected in any girl presenting with an inguinal hernia. More commonly these children are diagnosed at the time of puberty with amenorrhoea and lack of pubic or axillary hair. Because some testosterone and DHT is converted to oestrogen in peripheral tissues, the elevated levels of these hormones produced at puberty often results in adequate oestrogen levels for breast development.)

Case 4

This child has aniridia and ambiguous genitalia. WAGR syndrome incorporates Wilms' tumour, Aniridia, Genital abnormalities and Retardation. Denys–Drash syndrome comprises genital abnormalities, risk of Wilms' tumour and nephropathy; 30% of spontaneous cases of aniridia develop Wilms' tumour. A shared genetic locus for increased risk of Wilms' tumour, aniridia and some genital abnormalities exists at 11p13.

Case 5

This child has presented in addisonian crisis. His genitalia are described as normal except for micropenis and this should alert one to the possibility of hypogonadotrophic hypogonadism. Together, these findings could be explained by panhypopituitarism. 3β-Hydroxysteroid dehydrogenase deficiency is a rare form of congenital adrenal hyperplasia that blocks production of sex steroid, cortisol and aldosterone production. This presents with ambiguous genitalia rather than micropenis together with the risk of addisonian crisis, and is a second possibility in this case.

Case 6

XY undervirilised males may show great variation in the degree of development of both internal and external genitalia. The presence of a descended gonad, with evidence of internal female structures together with somatic features of Turner's syndrome strongly suggests a diagnosis of mixed gonadal dysgenesis) The karyotype is 45X/46XY mosaicism and two-thirds of cases will have some of the somatic manifestations associated with Turner's syndrome. Pure gonadal dysgenesis has no somatic manifestations. This presents with ambiguous genitalia rather than isolated micropenis.

Congenital adrenal hyperplasia

Enzyme deficiency	Male undervirilisation	Female virilisation	Salt loss	Hypertension
3β-Hydroxysteroid dehydrogenase deficiency	+	+/–	+	–
17α-Hydroxylase	+		–	±
21α-Hydroxylase		+	+	–
11β-Hydroxylase		+	–	±

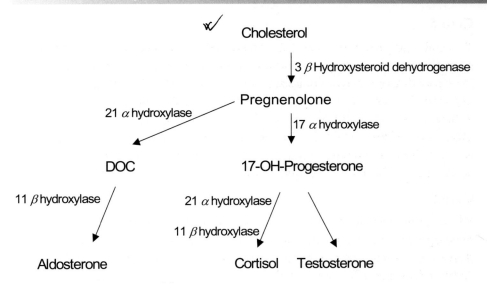

Outline of adrenal steroid biosynthesis

QUESTION 12

You are called to help with the management of a premature baby born at 26 weeks gestation. The baby was born by NVD after spontaneous onset of premature labour. The pregnancy had been uneventful until labour. Labour had commenced after spontaneous rupture of membranes 28 hours prior to delivery. The baby was initially cyanosed and apnoeic, with a heart rate of 70 bpm. Apgar score was 4 at 1 minute and the baby was electively intubated. Heart rate and colour improved rapidly. He was transferred to NICU and is now 45 minutes old.

12.1 What are the two most important findings on this X-ray?

. . . .

. . . .

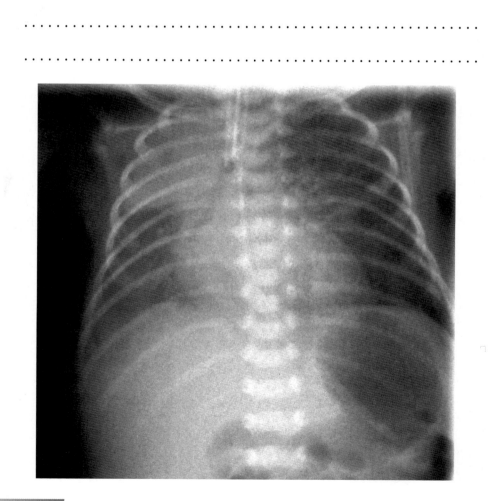

12.2 What two immediate interventions are necessary?

. . . .

. . . .

Ventilation remains difficult despite adequate sedation. At 4 hours of age there is a sudden increase in oxygen requirement.

CMV	P27/4 MAP 15, IT 0.34, RR 60, FiO_2 0.8, O_2 sats 80%
Arterial blood gas:	
pH:	7.1
pCO_2:	7.1 kPa
pO_2:	4 kPa
HCO_3^-:	16
BE:	−8

12.3 What does the arterial blood gas show?

- [ ] A Metabolic acidosis, adequate oxygenation
- [ ] B Respiratory acidosis with compensatory metabolic alkalosis
- [ ] C Mixed metabolic and respiratory acidosis, adequate oxygenation
- [ ] D Respiratory acidosis, adequate oxygenation
- [ ] E Inadequate ventilation, inadequate oxygenation, metabolic acidosis

12.4 What one test would you do immediately?

. . . .

The patient is stabilized over the next two hours. During this period he requires re-intubation.

12.5 What size endotracheal tube would you use?

- [ ] A 2.0
- [ ] B 2.5
- [ ] C 3.0
- [ ] D 3.5
- [ ] E 4.0
- [ ] F 4.5

12.6 How far would you insert the ETT before checking for equal air entry?

- ☐ A 4 cm
- ☐ B 6 cm
- ☐ C 8 cm
- ☐ D 10 cm
- ☐ E 12 cm

12.7 Which SEVEN of the following statements regarding this X-ray are appropriate?

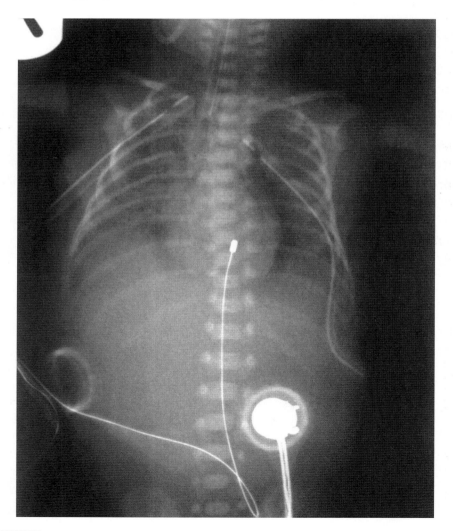

☐ A The ET tube is in the correct position
☐ B The ET tube is in the incorrect position
☐ C The NG tube is in the correct position
☐ D The NG tube is in the incorrect position
☐ E The UAC is in the correct position
☐ F The UAC is in the incorrect position
☐ G The UVC is in the correct position
☐ H The UVC is in the incorrect position
☐ I Bilateral chest drains are in situ
☐ J There is a tension pneumothorax
☐ K There is a pneumomediastinum
☐ L There is surgical emphysema
☐ M There is atelectasis
☐ N There is cardiomegaly

At 8 hours of age ventilation remains difficult. Current ventilatory settings are:

CMV   P 25/4 MAP 15, IT 0.34, RR 50, FiO_2 0.7, O_2 sats 94%
Arterial blood gas:
pH: 7.22
pCO_2:   8.5 kPa
pO_2:   7.0 kPa
HCO_3:   22
BE: −3

12.8 How do you interpret the arterial blood gas

☐ A Metabolic acidosis, adequate oxygenation
☐ B Respiratory acidosis with compensatory metabolic alkalosis
☐ C Mixed metabolic and respiratory acidosis, adequate oxygenation
☐ D Respiratory acidosis, adequate oxygenation
☐ E Inadequate ventilation, inadequate oxygenation, metabolic acidosis

12.9 What is the oxygenation index calculated on his latest gas (NB 1 kPa = 7.5 mmHg)?

- [ ] A 20
- [ ] B 22
- [ ] C 24
- [ ] D 26
- [ ] E 28
- [ ] F 30
- [ ] G 32
- [ ] H 34
- [ ] I 36
- [ ] J 40

12.10 What intervention would you make?

- [ ] A Increase ventilatory rate to 60, administer surfactant
- [ ] B Increase ventilatory rate to 60, increase Fio_2 to 80%
- [ ] C Increase inspiratory pressure to 28 cmH_2O, Increase ventilatory rate to 60
- [ ] D Increase PEEP to 5 kPa, Increase inspiratory pressure to 28 kPa, administer surfactant
- [ ] E Change ventilation strategy to high frequency oscillatory ventilation

At 8 days of age he remained ventilated. Over the following 72 hours, he developed an increasing oxygen requirement, became more tachypnoeic, less settled and tolerated feeds less well.

SIMV   P 18/4, IT 0.34, RR 30, Fio_2 0.4, O_2 sats 95%
Arterial blood gas:
pH :   7.27
pCO_2:   7.5 kPa
pO_2:   8.0 kPa
HCO_3^-:   17
BE: −8

Blood Pressure: 65/20

12.11 What are the TWO most likely causes for the increase in oxygen requirement?

☐ A Sepsis
☐ B Chlamydia pneumonia
☐ C Necrotising enterocolitis
☐ D Wilson–Mikity syndrome
☐ E Patent ductus arteriosus
☐ F Evolving chronic lung disease
☐ G Intraventricular haemorrhage

12.12 Given these findings what is your initial management?

☐ A Cranial ultrasound; chest X-ray; full septic screen, iv cefotaxime and gentamicin
☐ B Chest X-ray; full septic screen, iv cefotaxime and gentamicin
☐ C Chest X-ray; cranial ultrasound; full septic screen, iv cefotaxime and gentamicin; fluid restriction to 120 ml/kg per day
☐ D Full septic screen, iv cefotaxime and gentamicin and metronidazole
☐ E Fluid restriction to 120 ml/kg per day; indomethacin 0.1 mg/kg per day iv for 6 days
☐ F Fluid restriction to 120 ml/kg per day; await echocardiogram prior to starting indomethacin 0.1 mg/kg per day iv for 6 days

At 30 days of age he had an ongoing small ventilatory requirement.

12.13 Report on this chest X-ray taken on day 30 (4 points)

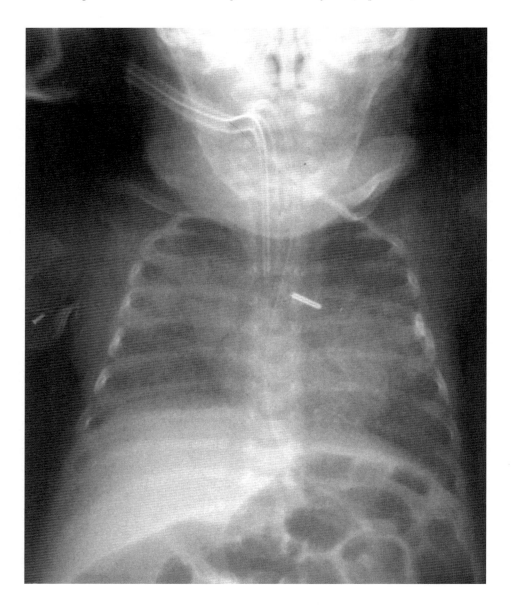

Answers to Question 12 are on page 108

ANSWERS TO QUESTION 12

12.1		Endotracheal tube in right main bronchus
		Right upper lobe collapse
12.2		Reposition the endotracheal tube (midway between clavicles and carina)
		Administer natural surfactant
12.3	E	Inadequate ventilation, inadequate oxygenation, metabolic acidosis
12.4		Transillumination of the chest
12.5	B	2.5
12.6	B	6 cm
12.7	A	The ET tube is in the correct position
	C	The NG tube is in the correct position
	E	The UAC is in the correct position
	I	Bilateral chest drains are in situ
	K	There is a pneumomediastinum
	L	There is surgical emphysema
	M	There is atelectasis
12.8	D	Respiratory acidosis, adequate oxygenation
12.9	A	20
12.10	A	Increase ventilatory rate to 60, administer surfactant
12.11	A	Sepsis
	E	Patent ductus arteriosus
12.12	C	Chest X-ray; cranial ultrasound; full septic screen, iv cefotaxime and gentamicin; fluid restriction to 120 ml/kg per day
12.13		ETT in situ in correct position
		Nasogastric tube in situ in correct position
		Patchy collapse and cystic overdistention consistent with bronchopulmonary dysplasia
		Visible clamp from surgically ligated PDA

Discussion

Surfactant therapy

Surfactant therapy is indicated at or soon after birth for any infant judged to be at high risk of developing respiratory distress syndrome (hyaline membrane disease). All babies born at < 30 weeks gestation should be given surfactant at birth if they need intubation. In practice babies at or below 30 weeks gestation are often electively intubated at birth, and prophylactic surfactant is given as soon as possible (RCPCH, 2000). Prophylactic surfactant given at or soon after birth has been shown to be more effective than rescue surfactant at 4 hours of age in preterm babies with RDS (Soll & Morley, 2000). There is a better outcome with two doses of surfactant rather than one, and a third dose is sometimes given in more severe RDS. Administration of surfactant for hyaline membrane disease reduces the incidence of pneumothoraces, pulmonary interstitial emphysema and death. The effect on the development of chronic lung disease, and on the frequency of intraventricular haemorrhage and patent ductus arteriosus is harder to define.

The position of the endotracheal tube is of utmost importance when surfactant is administered, as unilateral distribution may result in asymmetrical lung compliance with consequent overdistention and development of unilateral pulmonary interstitial emphysema (PIE).

Patent ductus arteriosus (PDA)

In term infants the ductus is normally functionally closed with the first 12 hours of life and anatomically closed with the first week. PDA is rare in term infants, more common in infants who have sustained hypoxia at birth and a frequent finding in very low birthweight infants requiring ventilation. Preterm infants tend to become symptomatic within the first 2 weeks of life as the pulmonary vascular resistance drops and a left-to-right shunt develops at ductal level. The signs of a patent duct are a new heart murmur, loud P2, bounding pulses, widened pulse pressure and an increasing oxygen requirement. Echocardiographic confirmation of clinical findings is recommended. A symptomatic PDA can often be managed successfully with fluid restriction. Indomethacin works to close the ductus by inhibiting the production of prostaglandin E1. It also affects other vascular beds, reducing both renal and gut perfusion. It can be given as a short course of three doses 12 hourly or a longer course once daily for 6 days. Renal biochemistry must be checked before each dose. The prolonged course has a greater success rate and less effect on renal function whereas gastrointestinal complications are comparable with both courses. Both the PDA itself and indomethacin affect gut perfusion and are risk factors for the infant developing necrotising enterocolitis (NEC).

Chronic lung disease (bronchopulmonary dysplasia)

This is defined as a persisting oxygen requirement together with chest X-ray changes at 28 days postnatal age or at corrected gestational age 36 weeks. X-ray changes of bronchopulmonary dysplasia when first described were staged into four grades ranging from uniform opacification to patchy collapse and cystic overdistention (as seen on page 106). With modern ventilation the changes seen are usually less dramatic with a less fibrotic, smoother opacification of the lung fields.

CLD is caused by multifactorial damage to the surfactant-deficient lung. Ventilation, infection, high concentrations of oxygen and in some studies hypocarbia and PDA have been shown to be associated with CLD.

Management aims to support the infant without causing further lung damage while at the same time optimising growth. Permissive hypercapnia aims to minimise ventilator-related lung injury. Babies may need sedation to achieve satisfactory ventilation even on synchronised ventilator modes as they often struggle against the ventilator (so called BPD spells). Low oxygen saturations increase the risk of pulmonary hypertension, whereas high oxygen saturations increase the risk of retinopathy of prematurity. Oxygen saturations of 90–93% are generally accepted.

Diuretics improve lung function in CLD. They can be useful in aiding extubation but have not been shown to reduce the total number of days in oxygen. The effect of diuretics is not sustained after withdrawal of treatment and consequently, if they are used on a long-term basis, they are generally continued in small doses until growth of new healthy lung tissue is adequate.

Steroids improve lung function in ventilator-dependent infants and have been used extensively in the past to aid extubation. However, poor neurodevelopmental outcome in association with dexamethasone treatment has recently been described with the relative risk of cerebral palsy at 2.32 (Halliday & Ehrenkranz, 2001). Steroids are therefore not currently recommended in the management of CLD unless the infant is unlikely to survive without them.

Oxygenation index (OI)

The oxygenation index is a measure used to define how effective the current ventilation strategy is at oxygenating the individual:

$$\frac{mean\ airway\ pressure\ (cm\ H_2O) \times FiO_2(\%)}{PaO_2\ (mmHg)}$$

A persistent OI > 25 can be used as an indication to change ventilation strategy from conventional to high frequency oscillatory ventilation (HFOV). A persistent OI > 40 is used as an indication for extracorporeal membrane oxygenation (ECMO).

Catheter and tube positions in the neonate

Endotracheal tube

Gestation (weeks)	Internal diameter (cm)	Length at lip (cm)
26	2.5	5–6 cm
28	2.5	6–7 cm
28–34	3.0	7–8 cm
34–38	3.0/3.5	8–9 cm
> 38	3.5/4.0	9+ cm
Position on CXR	midway between clavicle and carina	

Umbilical artery catheter

Weight of infant (g)	Size of catheter (FG)	
< 1500	3.5	
> 1500	5	
Position on imaging		
High	T10–T12	(level of diaphragm)
Low	L4–L5	(below renal vessels)

Umbilical venous catheter

Size of catheter	Position on imaging	
5 FG	Supradiaphragmatic IVC	T6–T10

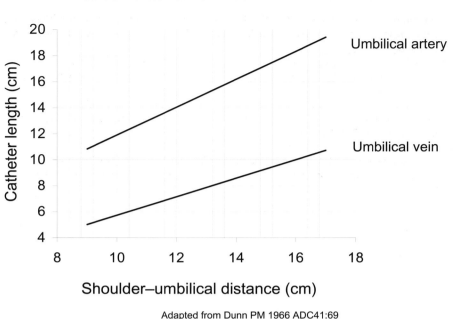

Insertion distance for umbilical catheterisation

Adapted from Dunn PM 1966 ADC41:69

Prophylaxis against RSV bronchiolitis (palivizumab)

Palivizumab is an effective anti-RSV monoclonal antibody that has been shown to reduce the rate of admission to hospital by 55% in premature infants < 6 months of age and by 39% in infants with CLD. However, as most premature infants with or without CLD will not require admission with RSV bronchiolitis even without treatment, the number of infants that need to be treated to prevent one admission to hospital is 17. There is consequently debate over the use of palivizumab in patients with CLD as there are clear financial constraints. There is, however, increasing evidence that treating patients with CLD with palivizumab not only reduces admission rates with acute RSV bronchiolitis but also reduces the use of health resources later in early childhood (Impact-RSV Study Group, 1998; Greenhough *et al.*, 2001).

References

Greenough, A., Cox, S., Alexander, J. *et al.* 2001. Health care utilization of infants with chronic lung disease, related to hospitalization for RSV infection. *Archives of Diseases in Childhood* **85**:463–8.

Halliday, H.L., Ehrenkranz, R.A. 2001. Early postnatal (< 96 hours) corticosteroids for preventing chronic lung disease in preterm infants. *Cochrane Database Systematic Reviews* Part 1:CD 001144–46.

Impact-RSV Study Group 1998. Palivizumab, a humanized respiratory syncytial virus monoclonal antibody, reduces hospitalization from respiratory syncytial virus infection in high-risk infants. *Pediatrics* **102**:531–7.

RCPCH 2000. *Guidelines for Good Practice.*

Soll, R.F., Morley, C.J. 2002. Prophylactic versus selective use of surfactant for preventing morbidity and mortality in preterm infants. *Cochrane Database Systematic Reviews* Part 2:CD 000510.

QUESTION 13

A 5-year-old Afro-Caribbean girl is seen in casualty with a 3-week history of progressive facial swelling, more noticeable first thing in the morning. She has become tired and irritable over this period and her parents are concerned that she is generally 'not right'. In the last 2 days she has had cold-type symptoms and her facial swelling seems to have increased. There are no other symptoms on specific enquiry except that she had a sore throat and fever for about 3 days, 4 weeks ago.

She was born at term after a pregnancy that was complicated by mild bilateral renal pelvicocalyceal dilatation detected on antenatal ultrasound. She was given prophylactic trimethoprim from birth until repeat renal ultrasound at 6 weeks of age showed complete resolution of the pelvicocalyceal dilatation.

Family history is unremarkable. She is sickle cell negative. She is fully immunised and her parents think she has had chicken pox previously. She required a blood transfusion 2 years ago when she was admitted to hospital after having been knocked down by a car. She is on no regular medication and has no known allergies. She has had recurrent tonsillitis over the last 2 years and is waiting to be seen in ENT outpatients regarding the potential need for a tonsillectomy. She has a history of intermittent constipation.

On examination she is alert, has generalized oedema and looks miserable. Heart rate is 100, blood pressure 90/45, respiratory rate 24 and temperature 36.2°C. Heart sounds are normal with no murmurs and breath sounds are vesicular bilaterally. Her abdomen is soft, non-tender, mildly distended and there is no palpable organomegaly. You manage to elicit a fluid thrill. ENT examination is unremarkable. Height 110 cm, weight 22 kg.

Initial investigations are as follows:

Haemoglobin:	11.8 g/dl
White cell count:	7×10^9/litre
Platelets:	298×10^9/litre
Sodium:	138 mmol/litre
Potassium:	4.2 mmol/litre
Urea:	2.2 mmol/litre
Creatinine:	45 μmol/litre
Cholesterol:	5.5 mmol/litre
Triglycerides:	2.2 mmol/litre
ALT:	24 IU/litre
Albumin:	18 g/litre
Bilirubin:	13 μmol/litre
Calcium:	1.8 mmol/litre
Phosphate:	1.4 mmol/litre
Varicella IgG:	negative
C3:	102 mg/dl (77–195)
ASOT:	1200 (120–160)
Urine dipstix:	Protein+4
	Blood+1

13.1 What is the likely diagnosis?

. . . .

13.2 Which FOUR investigations from those listed above support
this diagnosis?

. . . .

. . . .

. . . .

. . . .

✓**13.3** **Which FIVE further investigations are indicated?**

☐ A Hepatitis A serology
☐ B Hepatitis B serology
☐ C Hepatitis C serology
☐ D CMV serology
☐ E EBV serology
☐ F Measles serology
☐ G HIV screen
☐ H Complement CH50
☐ I Early morning urine protein/creatinine ratio
☐ J Antinuclear antibody
☐ K Antidouble stranded DNA antibodies
☐ L Chest X-ray
☐ M Urine microscopy and culture
☐ N Urinary sodium

13.4 **What is the most likely underlying pathology?**

☐ A Mesangiocapillary glomerulonephritis
☐ B Acute interstitial nephritis
☐ C Focal segmental glomerulosclerosis
☐ D Minimal change nephropathy
☐ E Proliferative glomerulonephritis
☐ F Membranous glomerulonephritis
☐ G Membranoproliferative glomerulonephritis
☐ H Post-streptococcal glomerulonephritis
☐ I Acute tubular necrosis
☐ J Crescentic glomerulonephritis
☐ K Henoch–Schönlein purpura nephritis
☐ L Berger's IgA nephropathy
☐ M Lupus nephritis
☐ N Goodpasture's disease

13.5 According to the modified ISKDC (International Study of Kidney Disease in Children) regimen for the treatment of this condition, what should be the *initial* treatment step?

☐ A Diagnostic renal biopsy and penicillin prophylaxis

☐ B Diagnostic renal biopsy, then empirical alternate day prednisolone 60 mg/m^2 28 days and penicillin prophylaxis

☐ C Single dose prednisolone 40 mg/m^2 per day 28 days and penicillin prophylaxis

☐ D Divided dose prednisolone 40 mg/m^2 per day 28 days and penicillin prophylaxis

☐ E Single dose prednisolone 60 mg/m^2 per day 28 days and penicillin prophylaxis

☐ F Divided dose prednisolone 60 mg/m^2 per day 28 days and penicillin prophylaxis

☐ G Alternate day prednisolone 40 mg/m^2 28 days and penicillin prophylaxis

☐ H Alternate day prednisolone 60 mg/m^2 28 days and penicillin prophylaxis

☐ I Penicillin for 10 days

☐ J Penicillin for 10 days, careful fluid balance, sodium restriction and antihypertensive medication if indicated

She is started on the recommended treatment. Her parents are very keen to know how effective the treatment is.

13.6 What is the likelihood that the recommended treatment will result in remission?

☐ A 30%
☐ B 40%
☐ C 50%
☐ D 60%
☐ E 70%
☐ F 80%
☐ G 90%
☐ H 100%

You are called to review her 24 hours into admission as she is complaining of abdominal pain, and when asked where it is worst she points to her umbilicus. She has felt nauseated all day but has not vomited, and has had one non-bloody loose bowel motion. She has not been coughing or become breathless. She has no urinary symptoms and has passed 100 ml of urine since admission. Her fluid balance chart shows her to be in slight negative fluid balance as she has not been keen to drink. She is alert. Her temperature is 36.3°C, heart rate 140, blood pressure 100/45, and respiratory rate 25. She is cool to touch. Her abdomen is non-distended. Central abdominal palpation is uncomfortable but she does not have rebound tenderness or guarding. Fluid thrill is present. Bowel sounds are normal. Her urinary sodium on admission was 8 mmol/litre.

13.7 What is the most likely cause of her abdominal pain?

- [ ] A Early appendicitis
- [ ] B Gastroenteritis
- [ ] C Intravascular volume depletion
- [ ] D Constipation with overflow diarrhoea
- [ ] E Spontaneous bacterial peritonitis
- [ ] F Urinary tract infection
- [ ] G Pneumonia
- [ ] H Acute pancreatitis
- [ ] I Iatrogenic peptic ulcer disease
- [ ] J Penicillin allergy
- [ ] K Volvulus
- [ ] L Acute tubular necrosis
- [ ] M Ascites

13.8 Which ONE option should be the first management step?

- [ ] A Surgical opinion
- [ ] B Stool culture
- [ ] C Frusemide 1 mg/kg
- [ ] D Frusemide 2 mg/kg
- [ ] E 10–20 ml/kg iv fluid bolus of 4.5% human albumin solution
- [ ] F 10–20 ml/kg iv fluid bolus of 20% human albumin solution
- [ ] G Frusemide 0.5 mg/kg

- [ ] H Abdominal ultrasound
- [ ] I Suppository/micro-enema followed by lactulose
- [ ] J Start trimethoprim at treatment dose
- [ ] K Chest X-ray
- [ ] L Intravenous ranitidine
- [ ] M Oral ranitidine
- [ ] N Refer to specialist renal unit
- [ ] O Abdominal X-ray
- [ ] P Measure amylase

✓13.9 **What does her urinary sodium concentration suggest in this context?**

- [ ] A She is developing diabetes insipidus
- [ ] B She has total body sodium depletion
- [ ] C Her kidneys are unable to conserve sodium
- [ ] D She has an element of hypoaldosteronism
- [ ] E She has a degree of renal failure
- [ ] F She is probably hypovolaemic
- [ ] G She has an element of SIADH
- [ ] H It is not helpful

After appropriate initial management her central abdominal pain subsides and her observations improve. You commence her on 30 ml/kg iv fluids to cover insensible losses and encourage her to keep trying to drink.

She begins to complain of more severe abdominal pain 24 hours later. She has had no further vomiting. Her fluid balance chart indicates a positive balance of 700 ml over the last 24 hours. Her morning urinary sodium was 20 mmol/litre. Her pulse is 110, blood pressure 85/50, RR 30 and temperature 38.7°C. On examination she is tachypnoeic without other signs of respiratory distress and her chest sounds clear. Cardiovascular examination is unremarkable. Her abdomen is non-distended. Abdominal palpation reveals increased non-specific tenderness with voluntary guarding and equivocal rebound tenderness. Urinalysis is 4+ protein, 1+ blood, 2+ leukocytes, nitrites negative.

13.10 What is the most likely diagnosis?

- [ ] A Acute pyelonephritis
- [ ] B Renal vein thrombosis
- [ ] C Rapidly progressing glomerulonephritis (RPGN)
- [ ] D Urolithiasis
- [ ] E Nephrocalcinosis
- [ ] F Iatrogenic peptic ulcer disease
- [ ] G Intravascular volume depletion
- [ ] H Renal artery thrombosis
- [ ] I Urinary tract infection
- [ ] J Spontaneous bacterial peritonitis
- [ ] K Pneumonia
- [ ] L GI perforation

This complication is managed appropriately and she recovers without further problems. Three weeks after discharge in remission she is in contact with varicella zoster when her brother develops unequivocal florid chicken pox.

13.11 What would you do next?

- [ ] A Commence aciclovir to reduce the severity of chicken pox should this develop
- [ ] B She should be given VZIG as she is immunosuppressed
- [ ] C She should be given VZIG now and then aciclovir if she later develops chicken pox
- [ ] D She should have her VZ antibody status re-checked
- [ ] E She should be given both VZIG and aciclovir as soon as possible
- [ ] F Stop her treatment

Answers to Question 13 are on page 122

ANSWERS TO QUESTION 13

13.1   Nephrotic syndrome

13.2   Albumin, urine dipstix, cholesterol, triglycerides

13.3   B   Hepatitis B serology

        C   Hepatitis C serology

        I   Early morning urine protein/creatinine ratio

        M   Urine microscopy and culture

        N   Urinary sodium

13.4   D   Minimal change nephropathy

13.5   E   Single dose prednisolone 60 mg/m^2 per day 28 days and penicillin prophylaxis

13.6   F   80%

13.7   C   Intravascular volume depletion

13.8   E   10–20 ml/kg iv fluid bolus of 4.5% human albumin solution

13.9   F   She is probably hypovolaemic

13.10 J   Spontaneous bacterial peritonitis

13.11 C   She should be given VZIG now and then aciclovir if she later develops chicken pox

Discussion

Nephrotic syndrome is characterized by heavy proteinuria (> 40 mg/m^2 per hour; early morning urine protein:creatinine ratio > 200 mg/mmol), hypoalbuminaemia, generalized oedema and hyperlipidaemia. Abnormal glomerular permeability causes protein loss in the urine with resultant hypoalbuminaemia. Plasma oncotic pressure is reduced with consequent fluid accumulation in the interstitium causing oedema. Lipids are high because the hypoalbuminaemia stimulates universal protein synthesis in the liver including lipoproteins, and also because lipid catabolism is reduced as lipoprotein lipase is lost in the urine.

The incidence of nephrotic syndrome is 2 in 100,000; 80% of children affected have minimal change disease (minimal change nephrotic syndrome – MCNS), which affects more boys than girls and tends to occur between the ages of 2 and 6 years; 10% have focal segmental glomerulosclerosis and the remaining 10% have mesangiocapillary glomerulonephritis or nephrotic syndrome as a secondary feature of a more complicated glomerular picture.

This last group includes postinfectious glomerulonephritis, hepatitis B infection, hepatitis C infection, lupus nephritis and Henoch–Schönlein purpura. These more complex conditions often give a mixed nephrotic/nephritic picture and should be suspected if the child is < 1 year or > 12 years, or if there are the additional findings of frank haematuria, hypertension or low plasma complement C3 levels (post-streptococcal disease; lupus).

This child has a pure nephrotic picture without hypertension or frank haematuria and is likely to have MCNS. The antistreptolysin titre is raised, but without features of nephritis and with a normal complement C3 level, post-streptococcal GN is unlikely. Similarly, although SLE is more common in children of Afro-Caribbean extraction, it usually occurs in adolescent females and the associated nephritis is characterised by a predominantly nephritic picture with a depressed complement C3 level.

Complications

The main complications of nephrotic syndrome are hypovolaemia, infection and thrombosis. Hypovolaemia and shock may occur despite fluid overload because of intravascular volume depletion due to reduced plasma oncotic pressure and maldistribution of extracellular fluids.

Infection risk is high in these children because they are on immunosuppressive therapy, immunoglobulins are lost in the urine, and ascites and oedema can act as a culture medium for bacterial infection. *Streptococcus pneumoniae* is the most common infective organism and may cause spontaneous bacterial peritonitis. Classic signs of peritonism may be absent or minimal in patients receiving corticosteroid therapy as illustrated in this case example. Children with nephrotic syndrome should be given Pneumovax® and receive penicillin prophylaxis until in remission.

There is an increased risk of thrombosis because the antithrombotic factors protein C, protein S and antithrombin 3 are lost in the urine, fibrinogen levels are elevated and these children are often relatively haemoconcentrated and immobile.

Treatment

MCNS is usually responsive to corticosteroids. As this group represents the majority of children with newly presenting nephrotic syndrome, empirical corticosteroid therapy is commenced without renal biopsy and histological confirmation in all children with nephrotic syndrome without atypical features. The ISKDC guidelines suggest single dose prednisolone 60 mg/m^2 per day for 28 days followed by 40 mg/m^2 on alternate days for a further 28 days. This should be completed even if remission is achieved, as there is evidence that duration of initial therapy may dictate likelihood and frequency of relapse. Those that respond are given the term 'steroid-sensitive nephrotic syndrome' (SSNS).

Relapse can be expected in 70% of children with SSNS. The first two relapses can be managed with prednisolone 60 mg/m^2 per day until clinical remission followed by 40 mg/m^2 on alternate days for a further 28 days. Up to 50% of children will have frequent relapses and are given the term 'steroid-dependent nephrotic syndrome'. They should be referred to a paediatric nephrologist. Maintenance prednisolone, levamisole, cyclophosphamide and cyclosporin are all used in the treatment of difficult steroid-dependent nephrotic syndrome.

The long-term prognosis for SSNS is very good with the vast majority of children achieving long-term remission before adulthood; 20% continue to have relapses into their twenties and thirties.

Reference

Holt, R.C.L., Webb, N.J.A. 2002. Management of nephrotic syndrome in childhood. *Current Paediatrics* **12**:523–606.

QUESTION 14

A 6-year-old boy is brought to casualty by his parents who are concerned that he is unwell and has developed a rash. The rash started on his trunk today and is now spreading over the rest of his body. Last night he felt hot, vomited twice and complained of a headache. He was restless overnight and stayed off school this morning. Over the course of today he has been vomiting and has seemed confused. His mother called his GP who came to see him this afternoon and noted a rash. He was given intramuscular penicillin and sent immediately to hospital by ambulance.

He is an otherwise fit and well boy and past medical history is unremarkable. He is on no regular medication, has no known allergies and was born at term with no perinatal complications. Development has been normal and he is fully immunised. There is no family history of note.

On examination he is drowsy with a Glasgow coma score of 11. Basic observations are: temperature 38.8°C, heart rate 120, blood pressure 160/100 and respiratory rate 30. Heart sounds are normal, capillary refill time is 4 seconds. Air entry is good bilaterally with oxygen saturations of 93% in air. Abdominal examination is unremarkable. He has a blanching macular rash over his trunk and limbs and occasional pinpoint petechiae on his face. He is photophobic and has meningism. Pupils are 4 mm bilaterally and react slowly to light. Fundoscopy is normal. He does not have decorticate or decerebrate posturing. Four-limb tone is normal and there are no false-localizing signs. Reflexes are slightly brisk with an equivocal plantar reflex bilaterally. He is receiving oxygen 10 litres/min, has two cannulae in situ and has already been given 80 mg/kg of ceftriaxone and a bolus of 20 ml/kg 4.5% albumin. The A&E consultant is present in the resuscitation room and has contacted the on-call general paediatric consultant and the paediatric intensive care unit.

14.1 From the list below which are the NINE most important initial management steps?

- [ ] A Lumbar puncture
- [ ] B Bedside glucose
- [ ] C Call anaesthetist to arrange urgent intubation and ventilation
- [ ] D Central venous access using internal jugular venous line
- [ ] E Peripheral arterial access
- [ ] F Full blood count, group and save

- ☐ G Coagulation screen, urea and electrolytes, calcium, magnesium, liver function tests
- ☐ H Start peripheral venous inotrope
- ☐ I Mannitol (0.25 g/kg) bolus followed by frusemide 1 mg/kg
- ☐ J Phenytoin 18 mg/kg over 30 minutes
- ☐ K CT scan brain then contact anaesthetist
- ☐ L 20 ml/kg 4.5% human albumin solution, repeated as required
- ☐ M Dexamethasone 0.4 mg/kg
- ☐ N Transfer to high dependency unit
- ☐ O Immediate MRI scan brain
- ☐ P 20 ml/kg 20% human albumin solution
- ☐ Q 3 ml/kg 20% human albumin solution
- ☐ R Venous blood gas
- ☐ S Sodium bicarbonate 1 ml/kg 8.4% over 20 minutes
- ☐ T CT scan brain once intubated and ventilated
- ☐ U Throat swab
- ☐ V Blood for PCR meningococcus
- ☐ W Chest X-ray
- ☐ X Blood culture
- ☐ Y Insert nasopharyngeal airway
- ☐ Z Central venous access using femoral venous line

14.2 Which SEVEN of the above are contraindicated?

. . . .

. . . .

. . . .

. . . .

. . . .

. . . .

. . . .

This boy was managed successfully and is much improved 4 days later. He developed seven petechial spots over his trunk soon after admission but these are now starting to fade. He remains on intravenous ceftriaxone and has been apyrexial for 24 hours. A blood culture taken on day one of admission has not grown any organisms, and a PCR to meningococcus is negative.

14.3 **What would you recommend regarding further antibiotic management?**

- [ ] A As both blood culture and PCR have not yielded an organism, stop the ceftriaxone
- [ ] B Take a further blood culture before deciding on the duration on antibiotic therapy
- [ ] C Continue at least 7 days of intravenous ceftriaxone
- [ ] D Change the antibiotic to an oral equivalent and then complete a 7-day course
- [ ] E Perform a lumbar puncture and, if the white cell count is normal, stop the antibiotic therapy

His parents are anxious to know what the risk of their daughter contracting this infection is, and whether she needs any preventative treatment.

14.4 **What is her risk if she does not receive antibiotic prophylaxis?**

- [ ] A 10%
- [ ] B 20%
- [ ] C 50%
- [ ] D 1%
- [ ] E 5%
- [ ] F 30–40%

14.5 Which THREE of the following require antibiotic prophylaxis?

☐ A School contacts
☐ B His 8-year-old cousin who stayed over last weekend
☐ C The nursing staff who looked after him whilst an inpatient
☐ D His brother
☐ E The GP who initially saw him
☐ F His parents
☐ G Prophylaxis is not required as this infection has not been proven

Answers to Question 14 are on page 130

ANSWERS TO QUESTION 14

14.1 B Bedside glucose

C Call anaesthetist to arrange urgent intubation and ventilation

F Full blood count, group and save

G Coagulation screen, urea and electrolytes, calcium, magnesium, liver function tests

I Mannitol (0.25 g/kg) bolus followed by frusemide 1 mg/kg

L 20 ml/kg 4.5% human albumin solution, repeated as required

M Dexamethasone 0.4 mg/kg

R Venous blood gas

T CT scan brain once intubated and ventilated

14.2 A Lumbar puncture

D Central venous access using internal jugular venous line

K CT brain scan then contact anaesthetist

N Transfer to high dependency unit

P 20 ml/kg 20% human albumin solution

Q 3 ml/kg 20% human albumin solution

Y Insert nasopharyngeal airway

14.3 C Continue at least 7 days of intravenous ceftriaxone

14.4 D 1%

14.5 B His 8-year-old cousin who stayed over last weekend

D His brother

F His parents

Discussion

This boy has presented with a rash, fever, shock and signs of raised intracranial pressure (ICP) (hypertension with relative bradycardia, altered conscious level, slowly reactive pupils and brisk reflexes). Although there are other possible diagnoses, by far the most likely is meningococcal septicaemia and meningitis. A rapidly appearing red, macular rash may precede the more classical petechiae in up to 40% of cases of meningococcal septicaemia. Any child presenting with an altered conscious level should have an immediate bedside glucose measurement. If the glucose is < 2.6, 2–5 ml/kg of intravenous 10% dextrose should be given immediately.

Initial resuscitation has been appropriate with volume replacement for compensated shock and intravenous antibiotics. Ongoing management of both his intravascular volume depletion with continuing fluid replacement and possibly inotropes, together with immediate management of his raised intracranial pressure are crucial.

Disseminated intravascular coagulation complicating meningococcal septicaemia should be anticipated. It is therefore important to take a full blood count, clotting and group and save at the initial presentation, as there is likely to be an early requirement for blood products (packed red cells, platelets, fresh frozen plasma and cryoprecipitate). Profound acidosis and electrolyte imbalance should also be anticipated and corrected.

The reasons for intubation and ventilation in this setting are then fourfold:

- facilitation of a safe CT scan procedure;

- anticipation of pulmonary oedema secondary to capillary leak syndrome and ongoing volume resuscitation;

- in the context of compensated shock, the energy expended in breathing for himself, unaided, may have a critical deleterious effect on cardiac output, and may significantly contribute to circulatory collapse; intubation and ventilation serves to take away this 'work' of breathing and therefore provide assistance in supporting his circulation;

- he has raised intracranial pressure and requires neurointensive care with ventilation, sedation and head-up nursing at 30° in the midline; optimising the pCO_2 to between 4.0–4.5 kPa is important as higher levels of pCO_2 will cause vasodilatation and increase intracranial pressure; conversely, cerebral vasoconstriction with a $pCO_2 < 4.0$ kPa will be detrimental and must be avoided.

Great care must be taken to prevent a critical drop in blood pressure on induction of anaesthesia. Rapid sequence induction should be undertaken using anaesthetic agents such as suxamethonium and thiopentone, together with atropine. Aggressive concomitant fluid administration (20 ml/kg 4.5% albumin) is also crucial in trying to preserve preload and maintain blood pressure.

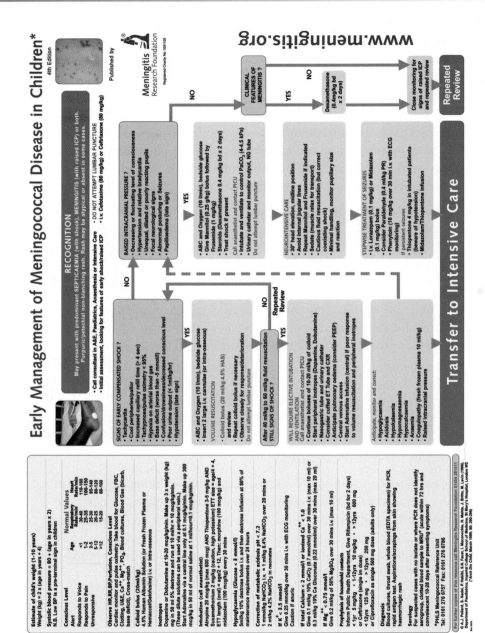

Early Management of Meningococcal Disease in Children*

4th Edition

Published by

Meningitis
Research Foundation
Registered Charity No. 1091105

www.meningitis.org

Reproduced by kind permission of the authors and the Meningitis Research Foundation

With reference to question 2, a lumbar puncture would be highly dangerous in the face of raised intracranial pressure. Central venous access is often needed relatively early but it is not one of the seven most important initial steps. If inotropes are required, dopamine should be started peripherally. In addition, the use of an internal jugular vein is contraindicated as it may increase intracranial pressure. Nasopharyngeal airway insertion may also increase intracranial pressure. A child in this condition should not receive a CT scan before his airway has been secured, and so option 'K' is contraindicated. This child is too unwell for HDU management and requires immediate intensive care.

Suspected meningococcal disease merits a full 7-day course of ceftriaxone. The antibiotic therapy should not be discontinued until the child has been apyrexial for at least 48 hours. Blood cultures are positive in approximately 50% of all meningococcal disease but fall to only 5% if the patient has already received antibiotics. Blood PCR for meningococcal DNA has a sensitivity of 88% and a specificity of 100%, and its use together with meningococcal culture has been shown to increase laboratory confirmation of clinically suspected cases by up to 35% (Hackett SJ et al., 1999).

The risk to a household contact of contracting the disease if they do not receive antibiotic prophylaxis is of the order of 1%. In pre-school children all household contacts in the preceding week should be offered prophylaxis. In children of school age, it should be offered to 'kissing contacts' or to overnight sleepers. The first-line recommended regimen is rifampicin twice daily for 2 days. Neither the ward nursing staff nor the GP require prophylaxis unless they have been in direct contact with pulmonary secretions, e.g. during intubation, mouth-to-mouth resuscitation.

References

Hackett, S.J., Carrol, E.D., Guiver, M. *et al.* 2002. Improved case confirmation in meningococcal disease with whole blood Taqman PCR. *Archives of Diseases in Childhood* **86**:449–52.

Pollard, A.J., Britto, J., Nadel, S., DeMunter, C., Habibi, P., Levin, M. 1999. Emergency management of meningococcal disease. *Archives of Diseases in Childhood* **80**:290–6.

QUESTION 15

As the paediatrician with the responsibility for hearing assessment in your trust, you are asked to consider a national proposal to screen all newborn babies for hearing loss using brainstem auditory evoked response (AER) testing. The introduction of this test into mainstream practice will signal the end of the community-based distraction test, which although cheaper to run is considered to be less effective than AER testing, the 'gold standard' in hearing testing.

To try and determine the true effectiveness of the distraction test, a pilot study has been carried out on 7500 infants aged 9–12 months, who have been tested using both methods. If the distraction test is proven to be as effective as AER testing, it will continue in your region to be the first line method of testing, and AER testing will be reserved for infants who fail the distraction test. The results of the pilot study are as follows:

	Auditory evoked response test		
	Passed	Failed	Total
Distraction test			
Passed	6960	80	7040
Failed	240	720	960
Total	7200	800	8000

15.1 What is the positive predictive value for the distraction test?

☐ A 90%
☐ B 75%
☐ C 88%
☐ D 97%
☐ E 99%

15.2 What is the negative predictive value for the distraction test?

☐ A 90%
☐ B 75%
☐ C 88%
☐ D 97%
☐ E 99%

15.3 What is the sensitivity value for the distraction test?

☐ A 90%
☐ B 75%
☐ C 88%
☐ D 97%
☐ E 99%

15.4 What is the specificity value for the distraction test?

☐ A 90%
☐ B 75%
☐ C 88%
☐ D 97%
☐ E 99%

You are then asked to interpret the results of an audiogram from a 7-year-old boy who has been referred because he is not doing well at school. He has no other specific symptoms, was well during infancy and has never previously been admitted to hospital.

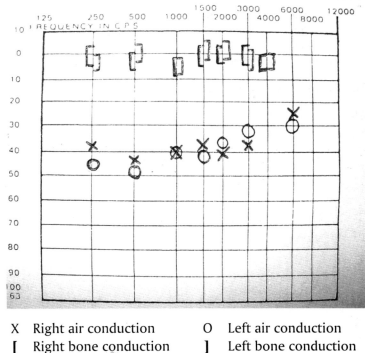

Key: X Right air conduction   O Left air conduction
        [Right bone conduction   ] Left bone conduction

15.5   What does the audiogram indicate?

☐   A   Bilateral sensorineural hearing loss
☐   B   Right conductive hearing loss
☐   C   Bilateral conductive hearing loss
☐   D   Left sensorineural hearing loss
☐   E   Normal hearing
☐   F   Left conductive hearing loss
☐   G   Right sensorineural hearing loss
☐   H   Mixed bilateral conductive and sensorineural hearing loss

15.6   Which of the following results would you expect from the
       Weber and Rinne tests if performed on this child?

☐   A   Right Rinne positive, Weber central, left Rinne positive
☐   B   Right Rinne positive, Weber to left, left Rinne negative
☐   C   Right Rinne negative, Weber central, left Rinne negative
☐   D   Right Rinne positive, Weber to right, left Rinne negative
☐   E   Right Rinne negative, Weber to right, left Rinne positive
☐   F   Right Rinne negative, Weber to left, left Rinne negative

15.7   Which of the following might account for the audiogram?

☐   A   Kernicterus
☐   B   Congenital CMV infection
☐   C   Congenital sensorineuropathy
☐   D   Chronic otitis media
☐   E   Previous aminoglycoside toxicity
☐   F   Previous head injury

Answers to Question 15 are on page 138

ANSWERS TO QUESTION 15

15.1 B   75%
15.2 E   99%
15.3 A   90%
15.4 D   97%
15.5 C   Bilateral conductive hearing loss
15.6 C   Right Rinne negative, Weber central, left Rinne negative
15.7 D   Chronic otitis media

Definitions

Positive predictive value: Indicates how likely it is that a patient with an abnormal test result (eg. failed distraction test) does actually have the disease in question (ie. is actually deaf).

Negative predictive value: Indicates how likely it is that a patient with a negative test result (eg. passed the distraction test) does not have the disease in question (ie. can hear).

Sensitivity: The ability of a test to identify true cases of a disease. Indicates the true positives with a disease.

Specificity: The ability of a test to identify those without the disease. Indicates the true negatives without a disease.

Discussion

In this case the brainstem auditory evoked response (AER) test is the gold standard test and indicates how many children can hear and how many are truly deaf. The results of distraction testing can thus be compared with those of the AER test to give an idea of how useful the distraction test really is.

The positive predictive value is a percentage that indicates how many children who are suggested as being deaf by distraction testing (960) are confirmed as actually being deaf by AER, 720/960, 75% (B), ie how accurate is a positive test result.

The negative predictive value is a percentage that expresses how likely it is that a child who passes the distraction test (7040) does actually have normal hearing on the basis of AER testing, 6960/7040, 99% (E), ie how accurate is a negative test result.

Sensitivity is calculated by taking the number of children who failed the distraction test (720) and expressing it as a percentage of those children who also failed the AER test and are actually deaf (800), 720/800 = 90% (A).

Specificity is calculated by taking the number of children who passed the distraction test (6960) and expressing it as a percentage of those children who also passed the AER test and so can definitely hear (7200), 6960/7200 = 97% (D).

The audiogram indicates that in both ears bone conduction is normal but air conduction is reduced. In the context of a 7-year-old underperforming at school, bilateral conductive hearing loss secondary to chronic otitis media is the most likely explanation. In the Rinne test, a child's ability to discriminate between air conduction and bone conduction is tested. Air conduction is tested by holding the tines of the fork parallel to the ear and approximately 2.5 cm (1 inch) away. Bone conduction is tested by holding the base of the fork firmly against the mastoid process. The child is then asked to compare the loudness of bone-conducted and air-conducted sound. Air conduction is usually heard better than bone conduction (Rinne positive). This finding is preserved in sensorineural deafness and reversed (Rinne negative) in conductive hearing loss.

In Weber's test, the tuning fork is typically held in the midline on the vertex of the skull and the child is asked to indicate whether he can hear the sound, and if so whether or not it preferentially lateralises to one side. Lateralisation does not occur with normal hearing or if a child has bilateral sensorineural or conductive deafness. Lateralisation occurs away from the affected side with unilateral sensorineural hearing loss and towards it with unilateral conductive loss. In the latter case this occurs because the middle ear increases its 'gain' in the context of conductive hearing loss. The results of these two tests can be summarised as follows:

Results

Right	Rinne	Weber	Left Rinne
A	Positive	Central	Positive
B	Positive	Left	Negative
C	Negative	Central	Negative
D	Positive	Right	Negative

Interpretation

A   Normal pattern, or mild/severe bilateral sensorineural deafness
B   Left conductive hearing loss
C   Bilateral conductive (or mixed) deafness
D   Left severe or profound sensorineural deafness

Kernicterus, congenital CMV infection, congenital sensorineuropathy, previous aminoglycoside toxicity and head injury all usually cause a sensorineural rather than a conductive pattern of deafness. There is nothing in the history or audiogram provided to strongly suggest any of these factors in this boy's deafness, and nor is this suggested by the audiogram provided.

Question 16

A 3-year-old boy is referred to the paediatric assessment unit with a 4-week history of cough. He first saw his general practitioner two weeks ago who prescribed a 1-week course of amoxycillin. His cough has persisted, and his mother has become concerned that he has become very tired and disinterested. There is no history of fever, shortness of breath or choking. He has become reluctant to eat and has become less interested in his toys. His stools are normal. There are no pets in the house. The family holidayed in Kenya 4 months ago, and he was well during this trip.

He was born at 32 weeks gestation and required ventilation for 24 hours, nasal CPAP for 3 days and oxygen therapy for a further 7 days. Since discharge at term he has been well and has been growing and developing normally. Until this illness he has had no respiratory symptoms. He has a brother aged 7 who has mild asthma. Both parents are well. He is fully immunized and has already had BCG vaccination, as his grandfather died 2 years ago, apparently from tuberculosis.

On examination he looks pale, but his skin is otherwise normal. He is alert. His pulse is 100, blood pressure 119/75 and respiratory rate 24. Examination of his neck demonstrates lymphadenopathy in the right anterior cervical and supraclavicular regions. Heart sounds are normal with no murmurs. All peripheral pulses are palpable. His work of breathing is normal, but on auscultation air entry is reduced in the right upper zone. Abdominal examination is unremarkable.

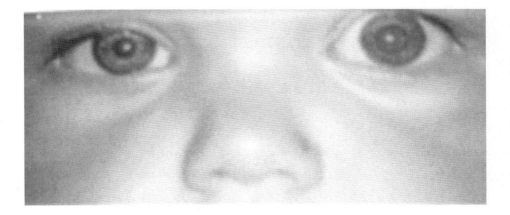

Both pupils are reactive to light, and fundoscopy is normal. Cranial nerves III to XII are intact, and he has normal four limb tone, power and reflexes. He has been walking around the assessment unit normally.

Initial investigations are as follows:

Haemoglobin:	7.8 g/dl
White cell count:	9×10^9/litre
Platelets:	342×10^9/litre
Ferritin:	262 μg/litre
Iron:	21 μmol/litre
Three thick and thin blood films:	no malarial parasites seen
Erythrocyte sedimentation rate:	53 mm/hour
C-reactive protein:	9 mg/litre
Sodium:	138 mmol/litre
Potassium:	4.2 mmol/litre
Urea:	2.2 mmol/litre
Creatinine:	45 μmol/litre
Alanine transaminase:	37 IU/litre
Albumin:	32 g/litre
Bilirubin:	18 μmol/litre
Calcium:	2.1 mmol/litre
Phosphate:	1.6 mmol/litre
Urinary Clinistix®:	Protein+1

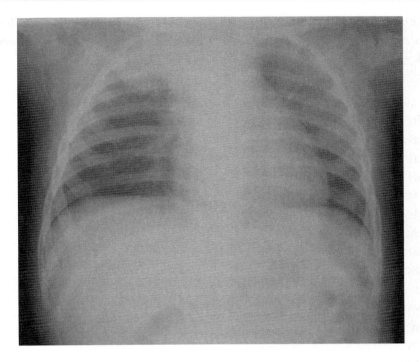

Chest x-ray

In view of his history he has a Mantoux test (10 U PPD) which is read at 48 hours:

Erythema: 4 mm   Induration: 6 mm

16.1 Which TWO of the following statements are correct?

- [ ] A   The Mantoux is negative and he probably does not have TB
- [ ] B   The Mantoux is equivocal and I would investigate further
- [ ] C   He probably has tuberculosis, particularly in view of the family history
- [ ] D   This test is not helpful in this child, as he is so unwell
- [ ] E   This reaction can be entirely attributed to previous BCG vaccination
- [ ] F   As the sum of the induration and erythema is 10 mm, this result is positive, and so he has tuberculosis
- [ ] G   Part of this response may be due to environmental mycobacterium
- [ ] H   As 25% of patients with later proven TB have a negative Mantoux test, this result does not mean he doesn't have TB

16.2   What is apparent examining his eyes?

- [ ] A   Right IVth nerve palsy
- [ ] B   Bilateral ptosis
- [ ] C   Right Holmes–Adie pupil
- [ ] D   Left Holmes–Adie pupil
- [ ] E   Right Horner's syndrome
- [ ] F   Right VIth nerve palsy
- [ ] G   Left IVth nerve palsy
- [ ] H   Duane's syndrome
- [ ] I   Left IIIrd nerve palsy
- [ ] J   Right IIIrd nerve palsy
- [ ] K   Left Horner's syndrome
- [ ] L   Left VIth nerve palsy

16.3   Which THREE of the following would be most useful in making a diagnosis and in further management?

- [ ] A   1/52 erythromycin to treat atypical pneumonia
- [ ] B   Gastric aspirate and early morning urine specimens, followed by commencement of antituberculous triple therapy
- [ ] C   CT of neck, thorax and abdomen
- [ ] D   Bronchoscopy
- [ ] E   Sweat test
- [ ] F   Echocardiogram
- [ ] G   Urine catecholamines
- [ ] H   Renal digital subtraction angiography
- [ ] I   Serum immunoglobulins G, A, M and E
- [ ] J   Lymph node biopsy
- [ ] K   Lung biopsy
- [ ] L   CT brain
- [ ] M   Angiotensin-converting-enzyme assay
- [ ] N   RAST for *Aspergillus fumigatus*

16.4   What is the most likely unifying diagnosis?

. . . .

Answers to Question 16 are on page 146

ANSWERS TO QUESTION 16

16.1 A   The Mantoux is negative and he probably does not have TB

     G   Part of this response may be due to environmental mycobacterium

16.2 E   Right Horner's syndrome

16.3 C   CT of neck, thorax and abdomen

     G   Urine catecholamines

     J   Lymph node biopsy

16.4   Neuroblastoma

Discussion

This boy presented with neck lymphadenopathy, a right Horner's syndrome and hypertension. Together with anaemia, high ferritin and the chest X-ray findings, neuroblastoma is the most likely diagnosis in this setting. Though falciparum malaria occurs in Kenya, repeated blood films are normal and foreign travel on this occasion is a red herring, as is the history of previous possible exposure to tuberculosis.

Neuroblastoma is a malignant tumour that may develop at any site of sympathetic nervous system tissue. Most cases arise in the abdomen, either in the retroperitoneal sympathetic ganglia or in the adrenal gland. One third of cases arise in the cervical, thoracic or pelvic ganglia. It is the commonest malignant tumour of infancy, the fourth commonest malignancy of childhood, and has an overall incidence of 1 in 100,000 with a median age onset of 20/12. It accounts for 8% of all childhood malignancy and 15% of childhood malignancy deaths. Associations include neurofibromatosis type 1 and Hirschsprung's disease.

Common presenting features are pallor, weight loss, an abdominal mass, hepatomegaly, bone pain and a limp. Less common but well-documented presentations include paraplegia, cervical lymphadenopathy, proptosis, periorbital bruising, skin nodules (blueberry muffin skin) and opsiclonus myoclonus, also known as the 'dancing eye syndrome'. The latter is a rare paraneoplastic manifestation attributed to autoantibodies specific for neural tissue. Calcification on abdominal X-ray should always alert one to the possibility of neuroblastoma.

Question 16.3 details the relevant initial diagnostic investigations. I-131-MIBG scintigraphy (chromaffin-tissue specific) detects non-skeletal metastases, and Tc-99m-MDP isotope scanning identifies bony metastases. Bone marrow aspirate may demonstrate classical 'rosette' formation of tumour cells.

The clinical extent of the disease, the patient's age and cytogenetic/molecular markers performed on tumour tissue (eg. amplification of the *n-myc* proto-oncogene) are together used to determine appropriate treatment. The International Neuroblastoma Staging System (INSS) is as follows:

- Stage 1   Tumour confined to the organ or structure of origin
- Stage 2   Tumour extends beyond the structure of origin but not across the midline, without (stage 2A) and with (stage 2B) ipsilateral lymph node involvement
- Stage 3   Tumour extends beyond the midline, with or without bilateral lymph node involvement
- Stage 4   Tumour is disseminated to distant sites (eg bone, bone marrow, liver, distant lymph nodes, other organs)
- Stage 4S   Children aged < 12 months who have dissemination to skin, liver or bone marrow, without bone involvement and with a primary tumour that would otherwise be stage 1 or 2. The importance of this distinction is in the fact that stage 4S has a better prognosis than stage 4, requires less intensive chemotherapy (in some cases supportive care only) and with time may regress spontaneously.

Based on *n-myc* amplification and clinical data, children can be divided into three prognostic groups, illustrated in the following table.

Risk	Clinical stage	*n-myc* amplification	Treatment	5-year event-free survival (%)
Low	1, 2 and 4S	Negative	Surgery alone	>90%
Medium	3, 4	Negative	'Mild' chemotherapy Surgery	80%
High	4, >1 year old; any stage and age with *n-myc* amplification	Positive	Chemotherapy Surgery Megatherapy Irradiation 13-*cis*-retinoic acid	30–50%

Adapted from: Castel, V., Canete, A. 2004. A comparison of current neuroblastoma chemotherapeutics. *Expert Opinions in Pharmacotherapeutics* 5:71–80.

QUESTION 17

Consider the following list of disorders:

A   Cushing's disease
B   Thiazide diuretic administration
C   Bartter's syndrome
D   Renin-secreting tumour
E   Conn's syndrome
F   Congenital hypertrophic pyloric stenosis
G   Cystic fibrosis
H   Anorexia nervosa
I   Recurrent vomiting (bulimia)
J   SIADH
K   Nephrogenic diabetes insipidus
L   Liquorice ingestion
M   Renovascular disease
N   Renal tubular acidosis type 1
O   Renal tubular acidosis type 2
P   Gitelman's syndrome
Q   21α-Hydroxylase deficiency
R   Salicylate ingestion
S   Paracetamol ingestion
T   Small bowel volvulus
U   Hirschsprung's disease
V   Chloride-losing diarrhoea

Case 1

A 4-week-old Asian boy is admitted to hospital with lethargy, poor feeding and weight loss. He was born at term to consanguineous parents, there were no perinatal complications and he had been thriving until 1 week ago, when he developed mild diarrhoea and occasional vomiting. This has persisted over the last 7 days, although he has continued to take fluids orally. On examination he is 5% dehydrated, lethargic but responsive. His pulse is 130, BP 70/45, RR 35, oxygen saturation 100% in air. Systems examination is unremarkable. His grandmother has mitral valve disease from rheumatic fever.

Tests show:

Na:	126 mmol/litre
K:	2.1 mmol/litre
Chloride:	80 mmol/litre
Urea:	4.2 mmol/litre
Creatinine:	35 μmol/litre
HCO_3^-	42 mmol/litre
Glucose:	7.8 mmol/litre
Urinary chloride:	20 mmol/litre

17.1   From the list of disorders, what are the TWO most likely diagnoses?

. . . .

. . . .

Case 2

A 5-week-old girl is admitted to hospital with a 1-week history of non-bilious vomiting described by her mother as projectile on occasion. She has had no diarrhoea. On examination she is 10% dehydrated with increased skin turgor and a depressed fontanelle. Pulse 160, RR 30, BP 60/40, oxygen saturations 95% in air. Systems examination is unremarkable. Test feed is negative.

Tests show:

Na:	131 mmol/litre
K:	2.3 mmol/litre
Chloride:	82 mmol/litre
Urea:	3.2 mmol/litre
Creatinine:	21 μmol/litre
HCO_3^-:	45 mmol/litre
Glucose:	5.6 mmol/litre
Urinary chloride:	10 mmol/litre

17.2   From the list of disorders what are the THREE possible diagnoses?

. . . .

. . . .

. . . .

17.3 What is the most important immediate investigation?

. . . .

Case 3

A 14-year-old girl is admitted to hospital with lethargy and dehydration. Over the last week she has been attending school as normal and her parents have not noticed any signs of illness. On examination pulse is 60, blood pressure 110/60, respiratory rate 12 and oxygen saturations 97% in air. Height 50th centile; weight < 3rd centile. On examination she has lanugo and poor dentition. Systems examination is otherwise unremarkable. There is no significant family history except her father has mitral valve disease.
  Tests show:

Na:	131 mmol/litre
K:	2.5 mmol/litre
Chloride:	84 mmol/litre
Urea:	4.3 mmol/litre
Creatinine:	45 μmol/litre
HCO_3^-:	33 mmol/litre
Glucose:	6.3 mmol/litre
Urinary chloride:	> 20 mmol/litre

17.4 From the list of disorders what is the most likely cause for these findings?

. . . .

17.5 What TWO other conditions from the list of disorders may rarely explain these findings?

. . . .

. . . .

Case 4

A 13-year-old boy is admitted from clinic with a blood pressure of 140/110 for further evaluation. He is an otherwise well child with no previous medical history. He is completely asymptomatic. Height and weight are both on the 25th centile. P85, RR 12, oxygen saturations 98% in air. Systems examination including full neurological examination is unremarkable.

Na:	142 mmol/litre
K:	3.0 mmol/litre
Chloride:	80 mmol/litre
Urea:	4 mmol/litre
Creatinine:	70 μmol/litre
HCO_3^-:	36 mmol/litre
Urinary chloride:	> 20 mmol/litre
Urinalysis:	blood −, leukocytes −, protein −, SG 1020

17.6 From the list of disorders what are the FIVE possible diagnoses?

. . . .

. . . .

. . . .

. . . .

. . . .

Renin and aldosterone levels are both shown to be elevated.

17.7 From the list of disorders, what are the TWO possible diagnoses now?

. . . .

. . . .

ANSWERS TO QUESTION 17

17.1 B Thiazide diuretic administration
     C Bartter's syndrome
17.2 B Thiazide diuretic administration
     F Congenital hypertrophic pyloric stenosis
     G Cystic fibrosis
17.3   Abdominal ultrasound
17.4 B Thiazide diuretic administration
17.5 C Bartter's syndrome
     P Gitelman's syndrome
17.6 A Cushing's disease
     D Renin-secreting tumour
     E Conn's syndrome
     L Liquorice ingestion
     M Renovascular disease
17.7 D Renin-secreting tumour
     M Renovascular disease

Discussion

The causes of metabolic alkalosis can be divided into two main categories based on the urinary chloride concentration. Urinary chloride is the best marker of volume status in alkalosis and a low urinary chloride (< 10 mmol/litre) suggests the metabolic alkalosis will be responsive to volume replacement.

In congenital hypertrophic pyloric stenosis, there is profuse loss of hydrogen ions and chloride ions in gastric secretions. This causes hypochloraemic alkalosis and volume depletion. The renin–angiotensin–aldosterone (RAA) system is activated secondary to volume depletion and enhances sodium reabsorption in exchange for potassium and hydrogen ions in the distal convoluted tubule (DCT), with consequent hypochloraemic hypokalaemic metabolic alkalosis.

Most children with diarrhoea who develop a metabolic acidosis do so as a result of enteral bicarbonate losses. In chloride-losing diarrhoea there is a defect in intestinal chloride/bicarbonate exchange causing chloride losses in the stool. Hydrogen ions and potassium ions are also lost with consequent alkalosis and hypokalaemia. Again, hypokalaemia and alkalosis are exacerbated by the RAA response to volume depletion. Chronic volume depletion alone may cause hypokalaemic alkalosis although this is rare.

Infants with cystic fibrosis may lose significant sodium and chloride through sweat with consequent volume contraction. The RAA system is again activated with consequent development of hypochloraemic hypokalaemic metabolic alkalosis with hyponatraemia. This is called pseudo-Bartter's syndrome.

Patients with metabolic alkalosis and a high urinary chloride can be separated based on blood pressure. A normal blood pressure and high urinary chloride suggests Bartter's syndrome, Gitelman's syndrome or the use of loop or thiazide diuretics.

Bartter's syndrome is an inherited autosomal recessive renal tubular defect of the sodium potassium 2-chloride transporter in the ascending loop of Henle. With this defect there is loss of renal sodium and chloride together with water and this causes volume contraction, which activates the RAA system. As described above this causes hypochloraemic hypokalaemic metabolic alkalosis. Gitelman's syndrome is an inherited renal tubular defect of the sodium/chloride cotransporter in the DCT. It has similar consequences to Bartter's syndrome but is milder and usually presents later in childhood. Both of these conditions have an elevated urinary chloride and this helps distinguish them from pseudo-Bartter's syndrome where the urinary chloride is low. Hypercalciuria is usually present in Bartter's syndrome whereas hypocalciuria occurs in Gitelman's syndrome.

The sodium potassium 2-chloride cotransporter is the site of action for loop diuretics and the sodium/chloride cotransporter is the site of action for thiazide diuretics. Both of these diuretics can therefore mimic the biochemical changes described above, and care must be taken to consider late onset Bartter's syndrome or Gitelman's syndrome if there is suspicion of diuretic abuse in a teenager with anorexia nervosa. It is important to note that urinary chloride level is high while on diuretics but will be low when the patient stops taking the diuretics.

Those patients with metabolic alkalosis, high urinary chloride and elevated blood pressure should have renin, aldosterone and cortisol levels checked. Elevated renin and aldosterone suggests renovascular disease or a renin-secreting tumour. Normal or suppressed renin levels with elevated aldosterone suggests Conn's syndrome (adrenal adenoma or hyperplasia). Low renin and aldosterone levels suggest a non-aldosterone driven mineralocorticoid effect, which may occur in children with Cushing's syndrome, congenital adrenal hyperplasia (usually 21α-hydroxylase deficiency), and in excessive liquorice ingestion.

Metabolic alkalosis

Low urinary chloride (<10mmol/l)

Congenital hypertrophic pyloric stenosis
Pseudobarrter's syndrome
Thiazide or loop diuretic (discontinued or chronic)
Recurrent vomiting
Recurrent NG aspiration
Chloride losing diarrhoea

High urinary chloride (>10mmol/l)

Normal blood pressure

Barrter's syndrome
Gitelman's syndrome
Thiazide or loop diuretic (current)

Raised blood pressure

Excess mineralocorticoid

Renovascular disease
Renin secreting tumour
Primary hyperaldosteronism (Conn's syndrome)
Cushing's syndrome
Congenital adrenal hyperplasia
Liquorice ingestion

QUESTION 18

You are asked to review a 3-year-old boy from a travelling family who have just moved to the area. His GP reports severe eczema and a chronic cough, which has been refractory to treatment with salbutamol and beclomethasone inhalers. He was born at term by normal delivery with a birthweight of 2.7 kg. There were no perinatal complications except for a rash that he developed soon after birth and which lasted for several weeks. His skin is dry, itchy and excoriated and has been a problem since birth. He has been given countless creams for eczema. He has also had recurrent skin infections requiring antibiotics and has had skin abscesses surgically drained from his left axilla on two occasions. He was admitted to hospital aged 13 months with a septic arthritis of his left knee and again aged 2 with severe Haemophilus influenzae pneumonia. He has had a chesty cough for the last year that has persisted despite three courses of antibiotics. He has received all vaccinations. His father has asthma and is a smoker. An uncle on the mother's side of the family had similar skin problems and died in childhood.

On examination his height and weight are below the 0.4th centile. His skin is excoriated and lichenified particularly on the face, wrists, axillae and groins. He has palpable lymphadenopathy in his groins, axillae and neck, and his tonsils are prominent. He has no chest deformity. On auscultation he has good air entry bilaterally with persistent course inspiratory crepitations on the right side. There is no audible wheeze or prolonged expiration. Cardiovascular, abdominal and joint examination is unremarkable.

Blood test results from GP show:

Haemoglobin:	12.2 g/dl
White cell count:	14.5×10^9/litre
Neutrophils:	4.0×10^9/litre
Lymphocytes:	2.5×10^9/litre
Platelets:	150×10^9/litre
ESR:	8 mm/hour

List A

A   Acute infection
B   Chronic infection
C   Chronic aspergillosis
D   Cystic fibrosis
E   Atopy
F   Severe combined immunodeficiency
G   Chediak–Higashi syndrome
H   Hyper-IgE syndrome
I   Chronic granulomatous disease
J   Wiscott–Aldrich syndrome
K   Leukocyte adhesion defect
L   IgG subclass deficiency
M   Mannose binding lectin deficiency
N   X-linked hypogammaglobulinaemia
O   Acute myeloid leukaemia
P   HIV infection

18.1   From List A, which SEVEN conditions are unlikely given the history, examination and initial blood results shown?

. . . .

. . . .

. . . .

. . . .

. . . .

. . . .

. . . .

18.2 From List A, which are the THREE most likely diagnoses?

. . . .

. . . .

. . . .

18.3 Which EIGHT further tests from List B would you elect to do next?

. . . .

. . . .

. . . .

. . . .

. . . .

. . . .

. . . .

. . . .

List B
A   Chest X-ray
B   CT chest
C   Sweat test
D   Full white cell differential and blood film
E   Quantitative serum immunoglobulins and functional antibody titres
F   IgG subclasses
G   IgE
H   Iso-haemagglutinins
I   Neutrophil function studies for chemotaxis
J   Skin prick allergy testing

K   Complement studies (CH50)
L   Mannose binding lectin (MBL)
M   Nitroblue tetrazolium test
N   Skin swabs
O   Skin biopsy
P   Spirometry with histamine challenge
Q   Bronchoalveolar lavage
R   HIV serology

18.4   Which chest diagnosis do the X-ray findings suggest?

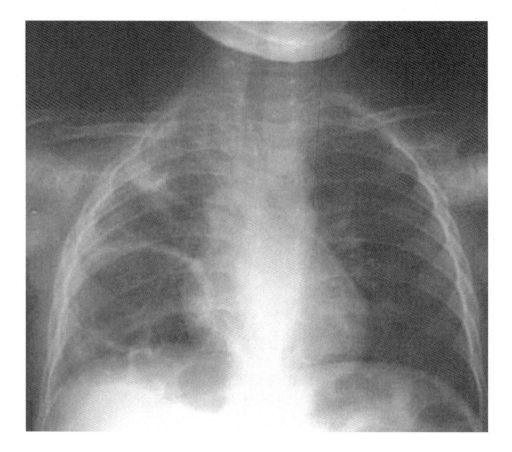

- [ ] A   Mediastinal mass
- [ ] B   Pneumothorax
- [ ] C   Congenital cystic adenomatoid malformation
- [ ] D   Congenital diaphragmatic hernia
- [ ] E   Bronchiectasis
- [ ] F   Pneumatoceles
- [ ] G   Immotile cilia syndrome
- [ ] H   Primary tuberculosis
- [ ] I   Post primary tuberculosis
- [ ] J   Bronchogenic cyst
- [ ] K   Cystic fibrosis
- [ ] L   Cardiomegaly
- [ ] M   *Pneumocystis* pneumonia

The result of his nitroblue tetrazolium test is negative.

18.5   Given this finding, what is the most likely unifying diagnosis?

- [ ] A   Acute infection
- [ ] B   Chronic infection
- [ ] C   Chronic aspergillosis
- [ ] D   Cystic fibrosis
- [ ] E   Atopy
- [ ] F   Severe combined immunodeficiency
- [ ] G   Chediak–Higashi syndrome
- [ ] H   Hyper-IgE syndrome
- [ ] I   Chronic granulomatous disease
- [ ] J   Wiscott–Aldrich syndrome
- [ ] K   Leukocyte adhesion defect
- [ ] L   IgG subclass deficiency
- [ ] M   Mannose binding lectin deficiency
- [ ] N   X-linked hypogammaglobulinaemia
- [ ] O   Acute myeloid leukaemia
- [ ] P   HIV infection

Answers to Question 18 are on page 160

ANSWERS TO QUESTION 18

18.1 A   Acute infection
   B   Chronic infection
   F   Severe combined immunodeficiency
   J   Wiscott–Aldrich syndrome
   K   Leukocyte adhesion defect
   N   X-linked hypogammaglobulinaemia
   P   HIV infection
18.2 G   Chediak–Higashi syndrome
   H   Hyper-IgE syndrome
   I   Chronic granulomatous disease
18.3 A   Chest X-ray
   C   Sweat test
   D   Full white cell differential and blood film
   E   Quantitative serum immunoglobulins and functional antibody titres
   F   IgG subclasses
   G   IgE
   K   Complement studies (CH50)
   M   Nitroblue tetrazolium test
18.4 F   Pneumatoceles
18.5 H   Hyper-IgE syndrome

Discussion

Hyper-IgE syndrome is a rare primary immunodeficiency characterized by recurrent severe staphylococcal infections affecting predominantly the skin, lungs and joints.

A distinct neonatal rash occurs in 75% of children, aiding early diagnosis in familial cases. Skin abscess formation is a problem from birth. All children develop a pruritic dermatitis but this is distinct from atopic dermatitis. Atopy is usually absent from the family history and asthma is uncommon. Persistent pneumatoceles typically develop as a result of recurrent pneumonia, with potential for superinfection and recurrent pneumothorax.

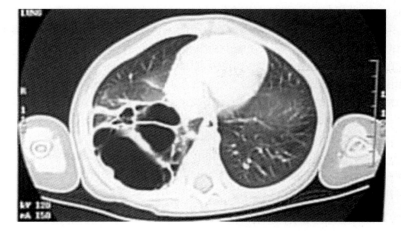

CT chest showing pneumatoceles

Laboratory findings include extremely high serum IgE concentrations and blood eosinophilia. Serum IgG, IgM and IgA are usually normal but functional antibody responses are poor. The underlying immune mechanisms responsible for hyper-IgE syndrome have not been fully clarified but are thought to be due to an imbalance in T-helper cell orchestration of the cell-mediated response. Recurrent infections may be due to excessive production of unprotective IgE with concurrent inadequate production of protective IgM and IgG. This group of patients also has variable defects in neutrophil function.

Recurrent invasive infection in childhood warrants immune system investigation. This child has had recurrent invasive pyogenic infections, which suggests a problem with humoral immunity. Recurrent skin abscess formation suggests a neutrophil defect. Severe immunodeficiency with prominent skin manifestations occur in hyper-IgE Syndrome, Wiscott–Aldrich syndrome, chronic granulomatous disease, the neutrophil granule defects including Chediak–Higashi syndrome, and in the leukocyte adhesion defects (LAD). Cyclical neutropenia should also be considered.

With reference to Question 18.1, severe combined immunodeficiency (SCID) is a rare extremely severe condition characterised by the absence of lymphoid tissue and lymphocytes, invasive viral infection, and PCP pneumonia in infancy. HIV infection can present in a similar way, but affected children will have palpable lymphadenopathy together with lymphopenia. Boys with X-linked hypogammaglobulinaemia are susceptible to pyogenic infections and recurrent pneumonia but also have a paucity of lymphoid tissue on examination. A low ESR makes chronic bacterial or fungal infection unlikely. Wiscott–Aldrich syndrome is characterised by atopic dermatitis, thrombocytopenia (15 × 10⁹/litre) with small defective platelets, and impaired humoral response to polysaccharide antigens (encapsulated organisms). These children may present with bloody diarrhoea early in infancy (Leukocyte adhesion defects present with recurrent skin infections, absence of pus but extremely high plasma neutrophil levels). (IgG subclass deficiencies may present with recurrent respiratory infections but this is usually later in childhood) Complement deficiencies present with recurrent invasive disease with encapsulated organisms and should be suspected in all cases of invasive meningococcal disease or neisserial septic arthritis.

Wiscott–Aldrich syndrome, chronic granulomatous disease, some variants of SCID, Bruton's hypogammaglobulinaemia, Duncan's lymphoproliferative syndrome and hyper-IgM syndrome are all X-linked immunodeficiency syndromes.

The management of hyper-IgE syndrome involves long-term prophylactic administration of antistaphylococcal antibiotics with aggressive treatment of invasive infection. Intravenous immunoglobulin should be administered to individuals with insufficient or absent functional antibodies. Thoracic surgery is indicated for chronic and superinfected pneumatoceles.

References

Erlewyn-Lajeunesse, M.D. 2000. Hyperimmunoglobulin-E syndrome with recurrent infection: a review of current opinion and treatment. *Pediatric Allergy and Immunology* 11(3):133–41.

Jhaveri, K.S., Sahani, D.V., Shetty, P.G., Shroff, M.M. 2000. Hyperimmunoglobulinaemia E syndrome: pulmonary imaging features. *Australasian Radiology* 44(3):328–30.

QUESTION 19

A 10-year-old is referred to the general paediatric clinic with a 6-month history of 'heart racing' accompanied by dizziness. Direct enquiry reveals no history of chest pain, shortness of breath, cyanosis or drop attacks. She is otherwise well and her weight is steady. Her only previous medical history dates back to the age of 3 when she had grommets inserted to try and reduce bilateral conductive deafness. Her mother's pregnancy was straightforward. She spent no time in the special care baby unit. A murmur was detected on her first-day check but had disappeared by day two of life and so no further action was taken. Family history is unremarkable. Her school performance has been poor this term. Her mother attributes this to bullying, which started after an episode of her becoming very breathless during a physical education lesson that she was unable to complete.

Examination is unremarkable. She is not dysmorphic and looks well. Pulses are all normal. Blood pressure in right arm is 98/65. Precordial examination is normal, with normal heart sounds and no murmurs. Respiratory and abdominal systems are normal. Neck examination is normal.

Initial investigations are as follows:

Haemoglobin:	13.9 g/dl
White cell count:	8.3×10^9/litre
Platelets:	282×10^9/litre
ESR:	9 mm/hour
Sodium:	141 mmol/litre
Potassium:	3.7 mmol/litre
Urea:	3.0 mmol/litre
Creatinine:	47 μmol/litre

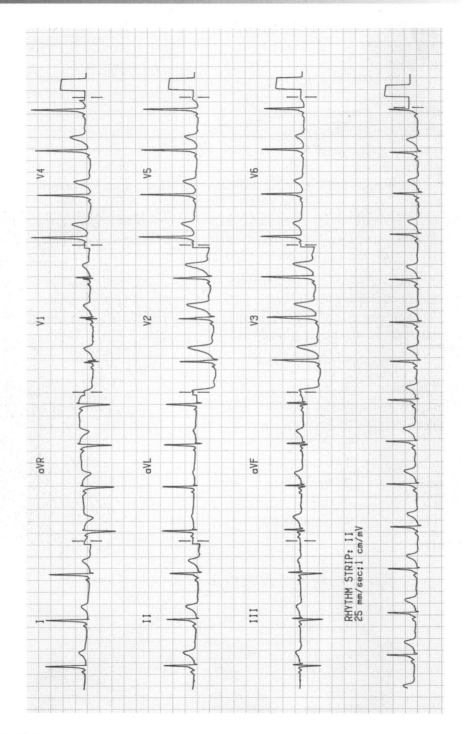

19.1   What abnormalities are apparent on this ECG?

- [ ] A   Short PR interval, J wave
- [ ] B   1st degree heart block, right ventricular hypertrophy
- [ ] C   2nd degree heart block (Mobitz type II)
- [ ] D   Delta wave
- [ ] E   1st degree heart block, narrow QRS complex
- [ ] F   None, this ECG is non-diagnostic
- [ ] G   2nd degree heart block (Mobitz type I)

Her GP has already ordered a chest X-ray.

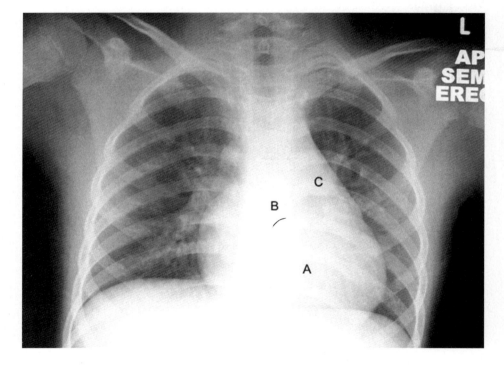

On this X-ray the position of three structures are marked 'A', 'B' and 'C'.

List A (Heart and mediastinal structures)

I   Mitral valve
II   Right ventricle
III   Left ventricle
IV   Pulmonary valve
V   Main pulmonary artery
VI   Left atrium
VII   Tricuspid valve
VIII Right atrium
VIII Thymus
IX   Superior vena cava
XI   Ascending aorta

For Questions '2', '3' and '4' refer to the above list.

19.2   The position of which structure is best indicated by 'A'?

. . . .

19.3   The position of which structure is best indicated by 'B'?

. . . .

19.4   The position of which structure is best indicated by 'C'?

. . . .

Whilst awaiting an outpatient paediatric cardiology opinion, she presents to casualty with a further episode of palpitations and dizziness. On examination she is tachycardic. Her blood pressure is 110/65. Examination of other systems is unremarkable. A rhythm strip is recorded during this episode:

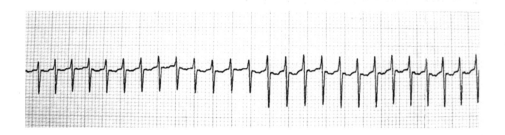

19.5   Which heart rhythm is apparent?

☐   A   Sinus tachycardia
☐   B   Ventricular tachycardia
☐   C   Sinus arrhythmia
☐   D   Supraventricular tachycardia
☐   E   Atrial flutter
☐   F   Atrial fibrillation
☐   G   2nd degree heart block

19.6   Which ONE of the following best describes your immediate management?

☐   A   Oxygen, vagal manoeuvres, amiodarone 5 mg/kg iv
☐   B   Admit for observation, offer strong reassurance, hearing test
☐   C   Oxygen, asynchronous shock 2 J/kg, 2 J/kg, 4 J/kg
☐   D   Oxygen, 12 lead ECG, chest X-ray, discuss with cardiologist
☐   E   Oxygen, synchronised DC shock 0.5 J/kg, 1 J/kg, 2 J/kg
☐   F   Oxygen, vagal manoeuvres, adenosine 50 μg/kg iv
☐   G   Oxygen, vagal manoeuvres, verapamil 0.1 mg/kg iv
☐   H   Admit for observation, thyroid function testing, echocardiogram
☐   I   Admit for observation

Following successful treatment for this acute episode she returns to clinic for further review. Clinical examination is now normal. She and her mother specifically ask whether it is safe for her to have children in the future, and what should be done should she become pregnant.

✓ 19.7 Which ONE of the following statements is true?

☐ A In light of this episode it would be dangerous for her to become pregnant

☐ B This episode does not increase her obstetric risk and no specific precautions are required

☐ C This condition can be familial and her children should have a 12-lead ECG in early life to exclude the diagnosis

☐ D This condition is inherited and associated with an increased risk of structural heart disease; fetal echocardiography is indicated

☐ E She should have an elective caesarean section at term

Answers to Question 19 are on page 170

ANSWERS TO QUESTION 19

19.1 D   Delta wave
19.2 II Right ventricle
19.3 VI Left atrium
19.4 V   Main pulmonary artery
19.5 D   Supraventricular tachycardia
19.6 F   Oxygen, vagal manoeuvres, adenosine 50 μg/kg iv
19.7 C   This condition can be familial and her children should have a
          12-lead ECG in early life to exclude the diagnosis

Discussion

The following table indicates ECG normal values in children:

Age	Heart rate	QRS axis	PR interval	QRS duration	V1 R/S ratio	V6 R/S ratio
< 1/12	95–145	75–180	0.08–0.12	0.04–0.08	0.5–inf	0.1–inf
1–2/12	110–180	35–135	0.08–0.12	0.04–0.08	0.3–1.0	1.5–inf
4–12/12	110–180	30–135	0.09–0.13	0.04–0.08	0.3–4.0	2.0–inf
1–3 years	105–170	0–110	0.10–0.14	0.04–0.08	0.5–1.5	3.0–inf
4–5 years	60–150	0–110	0.11–0.15	0.05–0.09	0.1–1.5	2.0–inf
6–8 years	60–130	−15–110	0.12–0.16	0.05–0.09	0.1–1.5	2.0–inf
9–11 years	60–110	−15–110	0.12–0.17	0.05–0.09	0.1–1.0	4.0–inf
12–16 years	60–100	−15–110	0.12–0.20	0.05–0.09	0–1.0	2.0–inf
> 16 years	55–100	−15–110	0.12–0.20	0.05–0.10	0–1.0	2.0–inf

Right ventricular hypertrophy		*Left ventricular hypertrophy*	*QT interval*
R wave > 20 mv in v1		R v5v6 > 26 mv	
Upright T waves in v1 at > 1/52 old, up to 4 years old		v1s + v5r > 40 mv	QTc=
Neonatal RS progression after 1/12 old		Q > 4 mv in v5 or v6	QT/$\sqrt{RR}$
Q wave in v1 in older children		T wave inversion in v5v6	
RAD for age			

The incidence of Wolff–Parkinson–White (WPW) syndrome is approximately 1.5 in 1000, although a majority never experience arrhythmias. It occurs in 9% of cases of Ebstein's anomaly. The typical ECG features are usually only seen when the affected child is not having a tachycardia, and occur as a result of pre-excitation of the ventricular myocardium through an accessory pathway. Anterograde conduction through both the atrioventricular (AV) node and the accessory conduction pathway cause fusion QRS complexes with the characteristic 'delta wave'. In SVT, an extranodal re-entry circuit is established with anterograde flow through the AV node (orthodromic conduction) and retrograde flow through the accessory pathway, which reaches the atrium and perpetuates the tachycardia. QRS complexes during an SVT are therefore normal in appearance. If during tachycardia rapid anterograde conduction occurs through the accessory pathway, and the retrograde re-entry pathway to the atrium is via the AV node (antidromic conduction), a wide complex tachycardia results. The potential then exists for more serious (potentially life-threatening) arrhythmias, particularly if atrial fibrillation occurs.

Management of SVT with no evidence of shock should begin with oxygen and vagal manoeuvres, and then proceed to adenosine if unsuccessful. Synchronised DC shock should be used only when there is evidence of cardiorespiratory compromise. In children known to have WPW syndrome, digoxin and calcium channel blockers should be avoided as they may precipitate ventricular arrhythmias. Propranolol and electrophysiological studies with ablation (where possible) are the mainstays of long-term management.

A working knowledge of normal cardiac and mediastinal anatomy is useful in day-to-day practice. The two figures illustrate the position of the main right heart structures (figure a) and the main left heart structures (figure b).

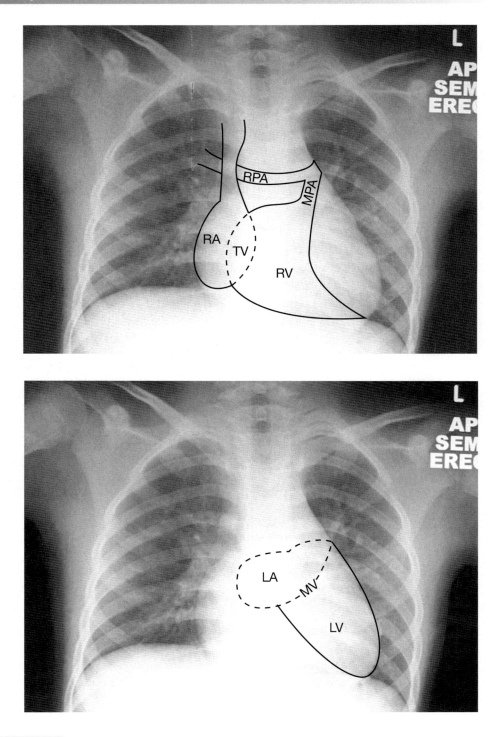

QUESTION 20

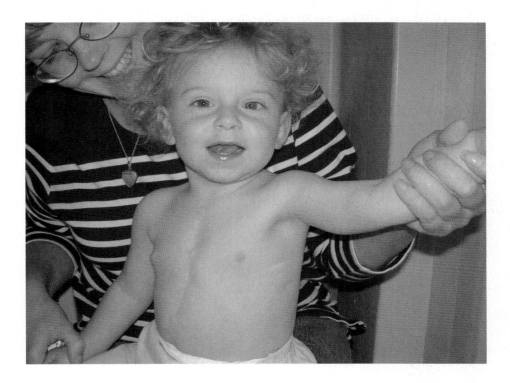

20.1. Which FIFTEEN of the conditions listed below can explain the above findings?

☐ A   Atrial septal defect
☐ B   Ventricular septal defect
☐ C   Ventricular septal defect and pulmonary stenosis
☐ D   Coarctation of the aorta and ventricular septal defect
☐ E   Coarctation of the aorta and aortic valve dysplasia
☐ F   Hypoplastic left heart
☐ G   Pulmonary stenosis
☐ H   Pulmonary atresia and ventricular septal defect
☐ I   Pulmonary atresia
☐ J   Critical pulmonary stenosis
☐ K   Tricuspid atresia with ventricular septal defect and pulmonary stenosis

☐ L Univentricular heart
☐ M Total anomalous pulmonary venous drainage
☐ N Partial anomalous pulmonary venous drainage
☐ O Atrioventricular septal defect
☐ P Patent ductus arteriosus
☐ Q Patent ductus arteriosus and ventricular septal defect
☐ R Swiss cheese ventricular septal defect
☐ S Tracheo-oesophageal fistula
☐ T Tetralogy of Fallot
☐ U Sequestration of left lung
☐ V Bronchogenic cyst
☐ W Congenital cystadenomatoid malformation and ventricular septal defect
☐ X Congenital diaphragmatic hernia
☐ Y Transposition of the great arteries
☐ Z Ebstein anomaly

Answers to Question 20 are on page 176

ANSWERS TO QUESTION 20

20.1 B   Ventricular septal defect
     D   Coarctation of the aorta and ventricular septal defect
     E   Coarctation of the aorta and aortic valve dysplasia
     H   Pulmonary atresia and ventricular septal defect
     I   Pulmonary atresia
     J   Critical pulmonary stenosis
     K   Tricuspid atresia with ventricular septal defect and pulmonary stenosis
     L   Univentricular heart
     M   Total anomalous pulmonary venous drainage
     N   Partial anomalous pulmonary venous drainage
     O   Atrioventricular septal defect
     Q   Patent ductus arteriosus and ventricular septal defect
     R   Swiss cheese ventricular septal defect
     T   Tetralogy of Fallot
     W Congenital cystadenomatoid malformation and ventricular septal defect

Discussion

Most congenital heart disease that cannot be managed medically is amenable to corrective or palliative cardiac surgery. Open-heart surgery is performed through a median sternotomy incision and is required for almost all valvular and septal surgery. The lateral thoracotomy incision is used for cardiac-related surgery, which does not require opening of the heart. A left thoracotomy is used in coarctation of the aorta, ligation of a patent ductus arteriosus, pulmonary artery banding in large left-to-right shunts and for insertion of an aortopulmonary shunt (usually a modified Blalock–Taussig shunt from subclavian artery to pulmonary artery). A right lateral thoracotomy can also be used for shunt surgery. The lateral thoracotomy is also used for lung surgery and for tracheo-oesophageal fistula repair (right side in normal situs). Uncomplicated ASD repair can be achieved through a submammary approach. Transcatheter device closure can be used for uncomplicated PDAs and ASDs, and is being assessed for use with muscular VSDs.

This child has both a median sternotomy scar and a left lateral thoracotomy scar.

(Any lesion that causes restricted right ventricular outflow (eg tricuspid atresia [K], pulmonary valve atresia [H, I], pulmonary valve stenosis [C, G, J], subvalvular pulmonary stenosis in tetralogy of Fallot [T], univentricular heart with associated pulmonary stenosis) may be severe enough to require an immediate palliative procedure to secure adequate pulmonary blood flow. This is usually achieved with insertion of an aortopulmonary shunt through a lateral thoracotomy incision. The exception is pulmonary valve stenosis where trans-catheter valvotomy is generally successful for all cases of simple stenosis and some but not all cases of critical stenosis. Corrective or further palliative surgery may then be performed at a later stage with open-heart surgery through a median sternotomy incision.) *

(Coarctation of the aorta is sometimes associated with a poorly developed left side of the heart, with associated defects including bicuspid aortic valve, subaortic stenosis and mitral valve abnormalities. Repair of a simple juxtaductal coarctation is possible through a left lateral thoracotomy incision, but repair of associated valvular lesions requires open-heart surgery (D, E).)

Cardiac conditions with large volume left-to-right shunting usually present with symptoms of pulmonary oedema and cardiac failure. If left untreated, pulmonary vascular resistance gradually increases and through vascular remodelling irreversible pulmonary hypertension ensues. Reversal of the shunt with right-to-left flow is the outcome (Eisenmenger's syndrome). Medical and surgical intervention is aimed at controlling heart failure and preventing pulmonary vascular changes, which may develop as early as 6 months of age. Large left-to-right shunts may occur across a VSD, PDA, ASD, AVSD, aortopulmonary window, in partial anomalous pulmonary venous drainage and in more complex cardiac disease such as univentricular heart syndromes without pulmonary outflow obstruction and truncus arteriosus. Large left-to-right shunts resulting from non-restrictive VSDs and AVSDs are usually repaired early in life but, if the child is either too small or has other associated cardiac lesions, early corrective surgery may be too risky and pulmonary artery banding to restrict the left-to-right shunt may be performed as a temporary palliative procedure. Swiss cheese VSD is the term given to multiple small defects in the muscular ventricular septum and these are often difficult to repair in infancy. Together these may create a significant left-to-right shunt, again requiring pulmonary banding with debanding and repair of the multiple defects at an older age.

Hypoplastic left heart is a term used to describe a spectrum of conditions relating to underdevelopment of the left side of the heart and ascending aorta. The left ventricle may be small or completely atretic. Pulmonary venous blood enters the left atrium and feeds to the right-sided circulation at atrial level. Mixing occurs and all systemic blood flow originates from the right ventricle passing through a patent ductus arteriosus to the descending aorta. Surgical intervention for this complex cardiac condition is in three stages (Norwood procedure I and II followed by a modified Fontan procedure). In the first stage, the single functioning right ventricle is employed to supply the systemic circulation and pulmonary blood flow is secured with a synthetic aortopulmonary shunt. In the second stage, systemic venous return from the SVC is connected directly to the pulmonary artery (Glenn procedure). Finally, systemic venous return from the IVC is connected directly to the pulmonary artery and the aortopulmonary shunt is disconnected (modified Fontan procedure). The result is that the systemic circulation is powered by the right ventricle and the pulmonary circulation is passive without a pumping chamber. Surgery for all univentricular heart conditions aims to employ the single functioning chamber as the systemic pump together with a passive pulmonary circulation.

QUESTION 21

A 6-month-old baby is admitted to the ward in early January with a 5-day history of worsening chesty cough, shortness of breath and poor feeding. He is afebrile with a pulse of 150, respiratory rate 65 and oxygen saturations of 80% in air, which respond well to mask oxygen. On examination he is dyspnoeic with subcostal and sternal recession, he has a hyperexpanded chest, reduced air entry bilaterally, palpable rattles and bilateral expiratory polyphonic wheeze with prolonged expiratory phase. Cardiovascular examination is otherwise unremarkable. He has a palpable liver 3 cm below the costal margin and small palpable lymph nodes in his groins. He has a florid rash of fine raised umbilicated lesions across his chest. He has oral candidiasis. He is estimated to be < 5% dehydrated. Head circumference and weight are both on the 0.4th centile. Major developmental milestones are normal but mother mentions that she is worried about his vision. The family are originally from the Sudan but moved to the UK 3 years ago. He was given one set of vaccinations at the age of 2 months.

21.1 What is the most likely diagnosis?

- [ ] A Pneumococcal pneumonia
- [ ] B Staphylococcal pneumonia
- [ ] C *Haemophilus influenzae* pneumonia
- [ ] D *Chlamydia* pneumonia
- [ ] E Measles
- [ ] F Adenoviral LRTI
- [ ] G Respiratory syncytial virus bronchiolitis
- [ ] H Parainfluenza viral LRTI
- [ ] I Influenza
- [ ] J SARS (severe acute respiratory syndrome)
- [ ] K Tuberculosis
- [ ] L Atypical pneumonia
- [ ] M Metabolic acidosis

21.2 What is your immediate management?

- [ ] A Admit to ward; oxygen
- [ ] B Admit to ward; oxygen, nasogastric feeds, CXR, nasopharyngeal aspirate for RSV (NPA)

☐ C Admit to ward; oxygen, iv fluids, CXR, NPA
☐ D Admit to ward; oxygen, iv fluids, CXR, NPA and blood cultures
☐ E Admit to ward; oxygen, CXR, FBC, UE, blood cultures, NPA, iv fluids, iv antibiotics
☐ F Transfer to PITU; Oxygen, CXR, FBC, UE, blood cultures, NPA, iv fluids, iv antibiotics
☐ G Transfer to PITU; oxygen, CXR, FBC, UE, blood cultures, NPA, iv fluids, iv antibiotics, Mantoux test
☐ H Admit to ward; oxygen, nasogastric feeds, nasopharyngeal aspirate (NPA) for RSV

21.3 From the description, what is likely cause for the rash on his chest?

☐ A Measles rash
☐ B Chicken pox
☐ C Impetigo
☐ D Exanthum subitum
☐ E Non-specific viral exanthum
☐ F Cellulitis
☐ G Erythema multiforme
☐ H Erythema nodosum
☐ I Molluscum contagiosum
☐ J Urticaria
☐ K Henoch–Schönlein purpura
☐ L Petechiae

He remains in hospital for the next 5 days with no significant improvement. Blood tests and a chest X-ray are ordered and he is commenced on iv cefotaxime. He deteriorates further and is admitted to PICU for ventilatory support.

Haemoglobin: 9.8g/dl
White cell count: 1.2×10^9/litre
Neutrophils: 1.2×10^9/litre
Platelets: 150×10^9/litre
Na: 145 mmol/litre
K   3.5 mmol/litre

Urea:	6.3 mmol/litre
Creatinine:	30 μmol/litre
Ca:	2.3 mmol/litre
ALT:	35 IU/litre
Bilirubin:	19 μmol/litre
ALP:	267 mmol/litre
Albumin:	35 g/litre
Total protein:	85 g/litre

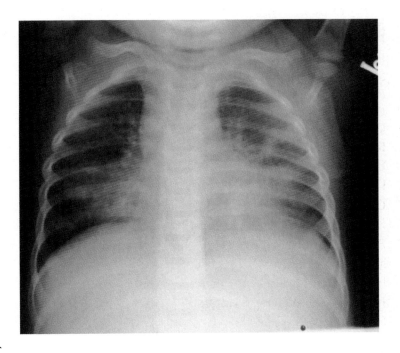

21.4 What is the likely causative organism now?

- [ ] A Respiratory syncytial virus
- [ ] B Adenovirus
- [ ] C Measles virus
- [ ] D Parainfluenza virus
- [ ] E Influenza virus
- [ ] F SARS coronavirus
- [ ] G *Pneumocystis carinii*
- [ ] H Cytomegalovirus
- [ ] I *Streptococcal pneumoniae*

☐ J *Staphylococcus aureus*
☐ K *Haemophilus influenzae*
☐ L *Chlamydia pneumoniae*
☐ M *Mycobacterium tuberculosis*

✓21.5 **Which other TWO organisms is it essential to exclude in this particular scenario?**

☐ A Respiratory syncytial virus
☐ B Adenovirus
☐ C Measles virus
☐ D Parainfluenza virus
☐ E Influenza virus
☐ F SARS coronavirus
☐ G *Pneumocystis carinii*
☐ H Cytomegalovirus
☐ I *Streptococcal pneumoniae*
☐ J *Staphylococcus aureus*
☐ K *Haemophilus influenzae*
☐ L *Chlamydia pneumoniae*
☐ M *Mycobacterium tuberculosis*

21.6 **What is the likely cause of the reported visual problems?**

. . . .

21.7 **What is the unifying diagnosis?**

. . . .

Answers to Question 21 are on page 184

ANSWERS TO QUESTION 21

21.1 G   Respiratory syncytial virus bronchiolitis
21.2 H   Admit to ward; oxygen, nasogastric feeds, nasopharyngeal aspirate
(NPA) for RSV
21.3 I   Molluscum contagiosum
21.4 G   *Pneumocystis carinii*
21.5 H   Cytomegalovirus
     M   Mycobacterium tuberculosis
21.6   *Mycobacterium tuberculosis*
21.6   CMV retinitis
21.7   AIDS

Discussion

PCP pneumonitis is a common first manifestation of HIV infection in infancy; 20% of infants infected through vertical transmission who do not receive prophylaxis will present with PCP pneumonitis in the first 3–6 months of life. This typically presents with increasing respiratory distress, profound hypoxia and a chest X-ray with ill-defined diffuse shadowing suggestive of interstitial pneumonitis. This presentation can easily be confused with RSV bronchiolitis during the winter.

CMV disease is another AIDS-defining illness that can present in the first year of life. CMV pneumonitis may co-exist with PCP pneumonitis and must be excluded. CMV retinitis is the likely cause for the visual problems described in this case.

Excluding *M. tuberculosis* is important and can be difficult as patients with untreated HIV may be anergic and unable to mount a response to the PPD/Mantoux test. Gastric lavage is probably the best diagnostic approach in this context.

Other findings in this case suggestive of HIV infection include lymphadenopathy and a description of molluscum contagiosum, which can be florid. The blood tests show a raised total protein and normal albumin suggesting raised immunoglobulins (IgG). This coupled with profound lymphopenia is highly suggestive of HIV infection.

Vertical transmission of HIV

Vertical transmission of HIV infection from an untreated HIV positive mother to her child can be as high as 30%. Intervention with antiretroviral therapy to the mother, elective caesarean section, antiretroviral therapy to the child and avoidance of breastfeeding reduces this transmission rate to < 1%. Antenatal screening coupled with the above intervention is dramatically effective in developed countries.

Nevirapine (a non-nucleoside reverse transcriptase inhibitor – NNRTI) given as a single dose to the mother during labour and to the child in the first 3 days of life reduces vertical transmission rates to 13%. It is an affordable, well-tolerated regimen that may help significantly reduce vertical transmission in less developed countries (Jackson *et al.*, 2003).

Diagnosis of HIV infection

Transplacentally acquired maternal HIV antibodies (IgG) persist for up to 18 months and do not represent HIV infection of the child. Diagnosis of HIV infection requires evidence of virus present in the infant – this can be done through HIV culture, p24 antigen tests or HIV PCR. HIV PCR is the test of choice and a common method of formal diagnosis is two positive HIV PCR tests at least 1 month apart with one test performed after the age of 3 months.

Children who are PCR-negative and IgG antibody-positive need to be followed up for at least 18 months to document loss of HIV antibodies (A positive HIV antibody test is diagnostic of HIV infection after 18 months of age.)

Staging of HIV infection

HIV infection is staged with reference to both clinical and immunologic criteria.

Clinical staging

N Asymptomatic

A Minimal symptoms
- Lymphadenopathy
- Hepatosplenomegaly
- Dermatitis
- Parotitis
- Recurrent URI

B Moderate symptoms
- Pancytopenia
- Systemic bacterial infection
- Candidiasis
- Cardiomyopathy
- Neonatal CMV
- Chronic diarrhoea
- HSV stomatitis, oesophagitis, pneumonia
- Herpes zoster
- Leiomyosarcoma
- Lymphoid interstitial pneumonitis (LIP)
- Nephropathy
- Nocardiasis
- Persistent fever
- Toxoplasmosis (congenital)
- Varicella (disseminated)

C Severe symptoms: AIDS defining disease
- Multiple bacterial infections
- Extrapulmonary cryptococcoses
- Cryptosporidiosis diarrhoea
- Oesophageal candidiasis
- Disseminated CMV
- Encephalopathy
- Persistent HSV
- Disseminated histoplasmosis
- Disseminated TB
- Atypical *Mycobacterium*
- *Pneumocystis* pneumonitis
- *Salmonella* sepsis
- CNS toxoplasmosis
- HIV associated malignancy (Kaposi's sarcoma, CNS lymphoma, B-cell lymphoma)

Immunologic staging

Degree of immunosuppression	<12 months CD4+/μl	%	1–5 years CD4+/μl	%	6–12 years CD4+/μl	%
None	>1500	>25	>1000	>25	>500	>25
Moderate	750–1500	15–25	500–1000	15–25	200–500	15–25
Severe	<750	<15	<500	<15	<200	<15

References

Jackson, B.J. *et al.* 2003. Intrapartum and neonatal single-dose nevirapine compared with zidovudine for prevention of mother to child transmission of HIV-1 in Kampala, Uganda: 18-month follow-up of the HIVNET 012 randomized trial. *The Lancet* **362**:859–68.

National AIDS Manual *http://www.aidsmap.com*

QUESTION 22

The picture below illustrates what a boy was able to draw when asked to 'draw a man'.

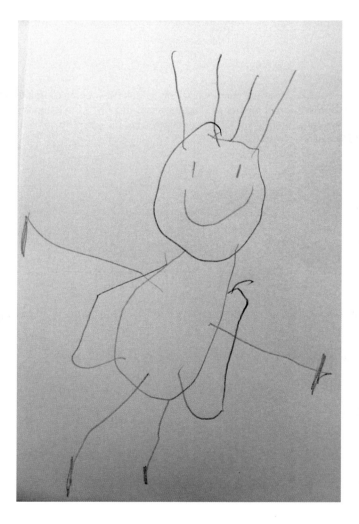

22.1 Select an age from the list below that most closely reflects this boy's cognitive ability as designated by the 'Goodenough–Harris' scale.

- ☐ A 3 years
- ☐ B 4
- ☐ C 5
- ☐ D 6
- ☐ E 7
- ☐ F 8

22.2 At what age (years) should a child of average ability be able to draw the following shape?

- ☐ A 2.5 years
- ☐ B 3
- ☐ C 3.5
- ☐ D 4
- ☐ E 4.5
- ☐ F 5
- ☐ G 5.5
- ☐ H 7
- ☐ I 8

22.3 At what age (years) should a child of average ability be able to draw the following shape?

- ☐ A 3 years
- ☐ B 2.5
- ☐ C 3
- ☐ D 3.5
- ☐ E 4
- ☐ F 4.5
- ☐ G 5
- ☐ H 5.5
- ☐ I 7
- ☐ J 8

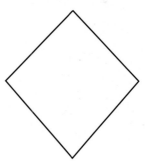

22.4 At what age (years) should a child of average ability be able to build the following structure with bricks?

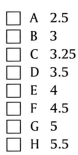 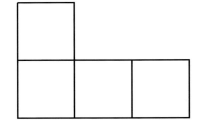

- [ ] A 2.5
- [ ] B 3
- [ ] C 3.25
- [ ] D 3.5
- [ ] E 4
- [ ] F 4.5
- [ ] G 5
- [ ] H 5.5

Answers to Question 22 are on page 192

ANSWERS TO QUESTION 22

22.1 C 5 years
22.2 F 5 years
22.3 I 7 years
22.4 C 3.25 years

Discussion

The Goodenough–Harris draw-a-man test was first devised in 1963 and can be used as a preliminary indicator of cognitive ability in children aged 3–8 years. As cognitive skills progress, drawing abilities also improve in detail and sex differentiation. Several studies have shown drawing abilities to correlate well with the results of more sophisticated assessments such as the Wechsler Intelligence Scale for Children-revised (WISC-R) and the Stanford–Binet Intelligence Scale (Abell, von Briesen & Watz, 1999; Tramill, Edwards & Tramill, 1980).

The child is asked to draw a man and then asked if he/she has finished before a score is assigned. The scoring system is as follows (1 point is given for each detail drawn):

 1 Head
 2 Neck
 3 Neck, two dimensions
 4 Eyes
 5 Eye details: eye brow or lashes
 6 Eye detail: pupil
 7 Nose
 8 Nose, two dimensions
 9 Mouth
10 Lips, two dimensions
11 Nose and lips (in two dimensions)
12 Chin and forehead
13 Bridge of nose
14 Hair I (any scribble)
15 Hair II (more detail)
16 Ears

17 Fingers

18 Correct number of fingers

19 Opposition of thumb (must include fingers)

20 Hands

21 Arms

22 Arms at side or engaged in activity

23 Feet (any indication)

24 Attachment of arms and legs (anywhere to trunk)

25 Attachment of arms and legs (at correct position of trunk)

26 Trunk

27 Trunk in proportion, two dimensions (length > breadth)

28 Clothing I (anything)

29 Clothing II (2 articles of clothing)

The child's total score (in this case 10) is then compared with a reference table that provides a typical score a child of a given age of average ability should achieve:

Age	Score (boys)	Score (girls)
3	4	5
4	7	7
5	11	12
6	13	14
7	16	17
8	18	20

The following illustrates when the drawing of specific shapes should be achieved:

12–18 months   Vertical scribble

2 years

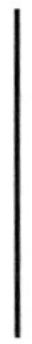

2–2.5 years   Circular scribble

2.5 years

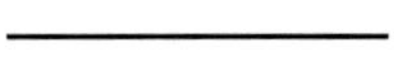

3 years

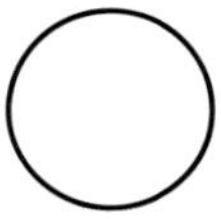

4 years

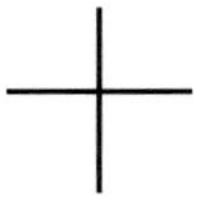

5 years

5.5 years

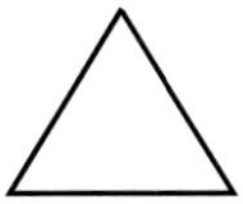

7 years

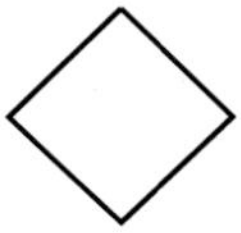

The milestones for building with bricks are as follows:

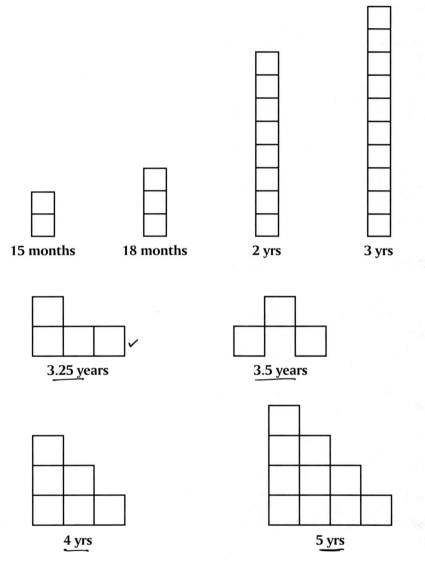

15 months 18 months 2 yrs 3 yrs

3.25 years 3.5 years

4 yrs 5 yrs

References

Abell, S.C., von Briesen, P.D., Watz, L.S. 1996. Intellectual evaluations of children using human figure drawings: an empirical investigation of two methods. *Journal of Clinical Psychology* **52**:67–74.

Tramill, J.L., Edwards, R.P., Tramill, J.K. 1980. Comparison of the Goodenough–Harris Drawing Test and the WISC-R for children experiencing academic difficulties. *Perceptual and Motor Skills* **50**:543–6.

QUESTION 23

You are asked to review a baby boy on the neonatal unit who is now 24 hours old. The neonatal team are concerned that he is floppy. Spontaneous onset of labour at 36 weeks gestation was complicated by failure to progress and fetal distress just prior to EMLSCS. The liquor became thinly-stained with meconium and the cardiotocogram (CTG) showed type I decelerations. Other than spontaneous premature labour there are no risk factors for neonatal infection. Booking serology was normal as was an anomaly scan at 20 weeks, and no concerns were raised regarding intrauterine growth. An ultrasound scan was performed at 32 weeks gestation because his mother reported reduced fetal movements. This demonstrated polyhydramnios, which persisted on subsequent scans. Mother was well in pregnancy and there is no history of consanguinity. This is her first pregnancy.

At delivery he had minimal spontaneous respiratory effort and received bag and mask ventilation before being intubated at 7 minutes of age. Cord gas pH was 7.21 (arterial) and 7.19 (venous). He has been on a ventilator since. Current settings are: peak pressure 16, positive end expiratory pressure 4, I-time 0.4 seconds, FiO_2 0.25. His most recent arterial gas was pH 7.41, pCO_2 4.7, pO_2 13.1, HCO_3^- 24. A chest X-ray taken at 4 hours of age showed clear lung fields and a normal heart size.

He is on a morphine infusion at 20 μg/kg/hr, 90 ml/kg/24 hours of 10% dextrose with supplementary sodium and potassium, and intravenous co-amoxiclav. The nursing staff are concerned that he has had very few spontaneous movements. No seizures have been noted. A cranial USS from today is normal.

The results of initial investigations are as follows:

Haemoglobin:	14.8 g/dl
White cell count:	13 × 10⁹/litre
Platelets:	412 × 10⁹/litre
Sodium:	135 mmol/litre
Potassium:	3.7 mmol/litre
Urea:	3.4 mmol/litre
Creatinine:	36 μmol/litre
CRP:	9 mg/litre
Alanine transaminase:	24 IU/litre
Albumin:	41 g/litre
Bilirubin:	73 μmol/litre
Calcium:	2.15 mmol/litre

Phosphate:	1.7 mmol/litre
Lactate:	1.4 mmol/litre
Ammonia:	47 μmol/litre
Urine dipstix:	protein +1

On examination his weight is 2.8 kg (10th centile) and head circumference 32 cm (25th centile). He is profoundly floppy with little spontaneous movement. Deep tendon reflexes are elicitable. On careful examination you note that he has distal contractures of the finger flexors. There is no hepatosplenomegaly. He is not otherwise dysmorphic.

23.1　On the basis of the information provided, which TWO of the following are the most likely possible diagnoses?

- [ ] A　Spinal muscular atrophy
- [ ] B　Hypoxic ischaemic encephalopathy
- [ ] C　Prader–Willi syndrome
- [ ] D　Congenital myotonic dystrophy
- [ ] E　Congenital myasthenic syndrome
- [ ] F　Neonatal adrenoleukodystrophy
- [ ] G　Congenital intrauterine infection
- [ ] H　Inborn error of metabolism

23.2　Which ONE of the following will be most helpful in distinguishing between these two possible diagnoses?

- [ ] A　Excluding maternal myotonia
- [ ] B　Congenital cataracts
- [ ] C　Bilateral cryptorchidism
- [ ] D　The resistance index on cranial USS
- [ ] E　The cord gas taken on delivery
- [ ] F　A family history of muscle disorders
- [ ] G　Brainstem auditory evoked response testing
- [ ] H　An inability to feed safely
- [ ] I　Evidence of renal failure and seizures
- [ ] J　Intracranial calcification seen on CT scanning
- [ ] K　The early development of acidosis, seizures and coma
- [ ] L　A patent ductus arteriosus
- [ ] M　Neonatal hepatitis

23.3 Which ONE of the following investigations would be most helpful in confirming the most likely diagnosis?

☐ A Very long chain fatty acids
☐ B DNA testing for spinal muscular atrophy
☐ C Edrophonium test
☐ D Electromyogram
☐ E Muscle biopsy
☐ F Anti-*Ach* antibody assay
☐ G DNA testing for congenital myasthenia
☐ H Creatine kinase
☐ I Electroencephalogram
☐ J Urine amino and organic acids

Answers to Question 23 are on page 200

ANSWERS TO QUESTION 23

23.1 D Congenital myotonic dystrophy
     E Congenital myasthenic syndrome
23.2 A Excluding maternal myotonia
✓23.3 G DNA testing for congenital myasthenia

Discussion

This case presents many of the differential diagnoses to consider when faced with a hypotonic newborn baby. This is not a typical history to suggest congenital infection. The presence of only thinly meconium-stained liquor, a lack of profound acidosis on cord blood gas and a normal lactate and urinalysis suggest this baby's problems are not as a result of perinatal hypoxia. This is further supported by the normal cranial USS (although this may be normal soon after delivery even in the face of significant perinatal hypoxia).

Gas exchange is good and the chest X-ray normal, making primary lung pathology unlikely. Neonates who require ventilation as a result of meconium aspiration typically have patchy changes on chest X-ray, with or without hyperinflation, and are usually significantly hypoxic.

The pertinent antenatal history in this case is that of polyhydramnios with reduced fetal movements, which taken together suggests this fetus might be weak and floppy and have difficulty in swallowing. After delivery, hypotonia, distal contractures and a lack of spontaneous movement are highly suggestive of a muscle or nerve disorder. Further history, clinical examination and investigation can narrow the differential diagnosis significantly. The presence of deep tendon reflexes does not support a ✳ diagnosis of spinal muscular atrophy. It is conceivable that a congenital myopathy could be the underlying diagnosis, but this diagnosis is not one of those listed and deep tendon reflexes are usually absent in this condition. Neonatal adrenoleukodystrophy usually presents with hypotonia and the early onset of seizures, though ventilator-dependence is not typical. Whilst an inborn error of metabolism is still a possibility, the preceding history, normal lactate, ammonia, liver function, urinalysis and a lack of acidosis together mediate against it. A lack of dysmorphic features mediates against Prader–Willi syndrome, as babies with this syndrome have a classical facial appearance (up-slanting almond-shaped palpebral fissures, narrow bifrontal diameter, and thin upper lip), small hands and feet, and bilateral cryptorchidism.

The history is consistent with a diagnosis of congenital myotonic dystrophy or congenital myasthenic syndrome. These two possibilities can be differentiated by establishing whether the mother has myotonia. In a child with congenital myotonic dystrophy who requires ventilation from birth, maternal myotonia will be unequivocally present. This is not a finding in a mother of a neonate with congenital myasthenic syndrome. Congenital myasthenic syndrome (CMS) is therefore the most likely diagnosis. This condition is not related to maternal myasthenia, and in contrast to maternally-derived transient neonatal myasthenia it is nearly always a permanent disorder without spontaneous remission. It is a channelopathy that occurs as a result of disordered function at the presynaptic, synaptic or postsynaptic level. The commonest CMS syndromes in children are as a result of mutations in the *Ach* receptor gene.

QUESTION 24

A 14-year-old boy is referred to A&E by his GP with a diagnosis of difficult asthma and acutely worsening shortness of breath. He had been relatively well until about 6 weeks ago when he developed a dry cough and difficulty breathing especially after exercise. Other than his 18-year-old brother, who had mild asthma when younger, there is no family history of note. The family have two cats and a budgie. Both parents smoke. He has received all his vaccinations, including BCG 6 months ago.

Despite being prescribed a salbutamol inhaler 6 weeks ago, he has also required two courses of oral prednisolone for his respiratory symptoms and this has helped his breathing on both occasions. He was started on beclomethasone 200 µg two puffs twice daily 3 weeks ago. Because of occasional fever, his GP took some blood tests and gave him a 3-day course of azithromycin 2 weeks ago.

24.1 What does this blood smear demonstrate?

. . . .

Room temperature   4°C

24.2 What infection does this finding commonly suggest?

☐ A Pneumococcal pneumonia
☐ B Staphylococcal pneumonia
☐ C *Haemophilus influenzae* pneumonia
☐ D *Mycoplasma pneumoniae*
☐ E *Chlamydia psittacci* pneumonia
☐ F Primary tuberculosis
☐ G Bronchopulmonary aspergillosis
☐ H *Bordetella pertussis*
☐ I *Pseudomonas aeruginosa*
☐ J *Burkholdaria cepacia*
☐ K Leptospirosis
☐ L Rocky Mountain spotted fever
☐ M Ricketsial disease

A full blood count showed:

Haemoglobin:	9.0 g/dl
White cell count:	28.4×10^9/litre
Platelets:	120×10^9/litre

Despite antibiotic treatment, his symptoms have progressed and his mother says that his breathing at night is becoming noisier and noisier. He has been sleeping sitting up in bed for the last 5 days.

On examination he is afebrile with a pulse of 95 and a respiratory rate of 40. Oxygen saturation in air is 93%. His chest is mildly hyperexpanded. Breath sounds are reduced bilaterally. He has a quiet biphasic stridor and intermittent expiratory wheeze. Cardiovascular examination is unremarkable. He has small mobile cervical lymphadenopathy and an injected oropharynx. He has a palpable spleen to 3 cm below the costal margin.

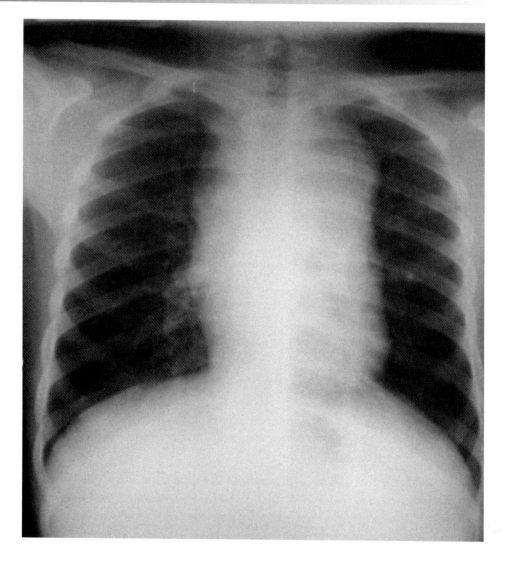

24.3   What is the most likely diagnosis?

. . . .

Answers to Question 24 are on page 206

ANSWERS TO QUESTION 24

24.1   Cold agglutinins

24.2 D *Mycoplasma pneumoniae*

24.3   T-cell lymphoblastic lymphoma (mediastinal mass)

Cold agglutinin disease is a subgroup of the autoimmune haemolytic anaemias and is characterised by the presence of red blood cell IgM antibodies that are more active at low temperatures. Cold agglutinin disease may be idiopathic or secondary to infections, particularly with *Mycoplasma pneumoniae* and EBV. It may also occur secondary to lymphoproliferative disease as in this case. The risk of intravascular haemolysis is increased with exposure to cold. The presence of cold agglutinins can be documented at the bedside by placing an EDTA sample of blood in the freezer for 10 minutes and looking for macroscopic evidence of agglutination. It is frequently positive in *Mycoplasma pneumonia* infection.

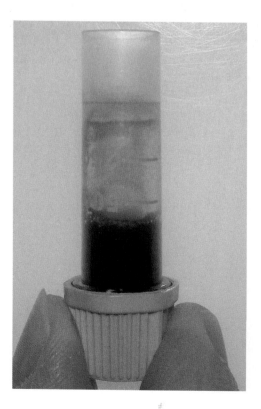

The presentation of non-Hodgkin's lymphoma (NHL) depends primarily on the site of disease. T-cell lymphoblastic lymphoma most commonly presents with an anterior mediastinal mass (50–70%). Local complications include compression of the intrathoracic airway giving rise to respiratory compromise and biphasic stridor, compression of the superior vena cava causing SVC syndrome, and pleural effusion.

Rapid growth and early dissemination are typical of NHL and consequently diagnosis, staging and initiation of treatment must be prompt. Tissue diagnosis must be made and can sometimes be difficult if the tumour is causing respiratory compromise, as a general anaesthetic may be impossible. Diagnostic material can be obtained from pleural fluid, peripheral lymphadenopathy, bone marrow, or CSF.

T-cell NHL and T-cell ALL represent a spectrum of disease. By definition, if there is > 25% bone marrow infiltration, the diagnosis is T-cell acute lymphoblastic leukaemia.

T-cell lymphoblastic lymphoma is exquisitely sensitive to steroid therapy, which will shrink a mediastinal mass rapidly. Tumour lysis syndrome is a common consequence of treatment, and with large mediastinal tumours it may even occur pretreatment. Lactate dehydrogenase is a marker of rapid cell turnover and is used to assess the likelihood of tumour lysis syndrome occurring on the initiation of treatment.

QUESTION 25

A 3-week-old baby is admitted with a 2-day history of poor feeding, fever and vomiting. She was born at term with no perinatal complications with a birthweight of 3.1 kg. Mother took early discharge at 6 hours. Progress with breastfeeding has been slow and she has not yet regained her birthweight. Family history is unremarkable.

On examination her temperature is 38.8°C, and she is jaundiced, floppy and sleepy. Observations are pulse 165, mean blood pressure 45 mmHg, respiratory rate 40 and sats 98% in air. Examination reveals 5 cm hepatomegaly, a full fontanelle, reduced four-limb tone but normal tendon reflexes. There is no rash and other systems examination is normal. Weight is 2.7 kg, head circumference 35 cm.

Her initial investigations are as follows:

Haemoglobin:	13.5 g/dl
White cell count:	24.2 × 10⁹/litre
Platelets:	41 × 10⁹/litre
PT:	20 s
APTT:	78 s
C-reactive protein:	131 mg/litre
Glucose:	1.4 mmol/litre
Sodium:	124 mmol/litre
Potassium:	4.2 mmol/litre
Urea:	6.0 mmol/litre
Creatinine:	47 μmol/litre
Bicarbonate:	16 mmol/litre
Bilirubin:	268 μmol/litre
ALT:	324 IU/litre
Albumin:	31 g/litre
Ammonia:	47 μmol/litre
Lactate:	1.9 mmol/litre

25.1 Having considered any specific investigation you may want to carry out, what is the best immediate treatment for the blood glucose of 1.4?

☐ A Repeat in 1 hour
☐ B 2 ml/kg bolus peripheral normal saline
☐ C 2 ml/kg bolus peripheral iv 0.45% saline/5% dextrose
☐ D 2 ml/kg bolus peripheral 4% dextrose/0.18% saline
☐ E 2 ml/kg bolus central iv 20% dextrose
☐ F 2 ml/kg bolus peripheral iv 10% dextrose
☐ G 2 ml/kg bolus central iv 50% dextrose
☐ H 10 ml/kg bolus peripheral normal saline
☐ I 10 ml/kg bolus peripheral iv 0.45% saline/5% dextrose
☐ J 10 ml/kg bolus peripheral 4% dextrose/0.18% saline
☐ K 10 ml/kg bolus peripheral iv 10% dextrose
☐ L 10 ml/kg bolus central iv 20% dextrose
☐ M 10 ml/kg bolus central iv 50% dextrose
☐ N Glucagon 0.04 mg/kg iv stat
☐ O Offer milk feed

The results of a full septic screen are as follows:

Chest X-ray:	Unremarkable
Blood culture:	No growth at 48 hours
Urinalysis:	Leukocytes 3+
	Nitrites –
	Protein 1+
	Blood –
	Bilirubin +
	pH 5
	Glucose –
	SG 1015
	Culture awaited
CSF:	Protein 1.7 g/dl
	Glucose 1.9 mmol/litre
	White cell count 87×10^6/litre
	Red cell count 8×10^6/litre

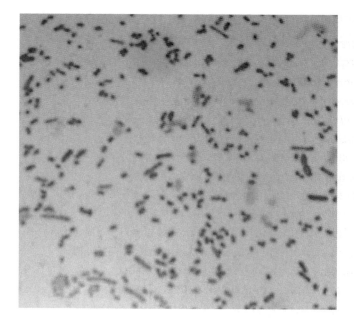

25.2   What does the CSF microscopy demonstrate?

☐   A   Gram-positive cocci in chains
☐   B   Gram-negative cocci in chains
☐   C   Gram-positive diplococci
☐   D   Gram-negative diplococci
☐   E   Gram-positive coccobacilli
☐   F   Gram-negative coccobacilli
☐   G   Gram-positive bacilli
☐   H   Gram-negative bacilli
☐   I   Gram-negative gonococci
☐   J   Mixed infection/possible contamination

25.3 Which organism is most likely present in the CSF?

☐ A *Listeria monocytogenes*
☐ B *Streptococcus pneumoniae*
☐ C *Haemophilus influenzae*
☐ D *Streptococcus agalactiae*
☐ E *Streptococcus viridans*
☐ F *Chlamydia pneumoniae*
☐ G *Neisseria meningitidis*
☐ H *Escherichia coli*
☐ I *Neisseria gonorrhoea*

25.4 What THREE conclusions can be drawn from the results of urine testing?

☐ A The low pH suggests low acidity
☐ B She has a mixed hyperbilirubinaemia
☐ C The urine is very concentrated
☐ D A UTI is unlikely as nitrites would usually be present in the urine
☐ E She has a purely unconjugated hyperbilirubinaemia
☐ F The low pH suggests high acidity
☐ G The urine is very dilute
☐ H She probably has a urinary tract infection (UTI)

25.5 Which of the following may be contributing to the hyponatraemia? (Any number may be correct)

☐ A Cerebral salt wasting
☐ B SIADH
☐ C Vomiting
☐ D Associated proximal renal tubular defect
☐ E Urinary tract infection associated tubulopathy
☐ F All of the above

She was started on intravenous cefotaxime and ampicillin, and nasogastric tube feeds at 150 ml/kg per 24 hours on admission; 6 days into this treatment there has been little discernible improvement in her condition. CSF and blood culture taken on admission grew the organism initially seen on CSF microscopy. Although her temperature settled after 4 days of antibiotics, she remains drowsy, continues to vomit, and is more jaundiced than previously. On examination she is now apyrexial, her fontanelle is flat, and her head circumference is 34.9 cm. Systems examination is otherwise unchanged from admission.

Repeat blood tests are as follows:

Haemoglobin:	13.6 g/dl
White cell count:	12×10^9/litre
Platelets:	47×10^9/litre
PT:	19 s
APTT:	77 s
Sodium:	129 mmol/litre
Potassium:	3.2 mmol/litre
Urea:	7.1 mmol/litre
Creatinine:	51 μmol/litre
Bicarbonate:	16 mmol/litre
Total bilirubin:	341 mmol/litre
ALT:	296 IU/litre
Albumin:	21 g/litre
Glucose:	2.1 mmol/litre
Urine:	Leukocytes –
	Nitrites –
	Protein 1+
	Blood nil
	Bilirubin +
	pH 5
	Glucose –
	Clinitest positive

25.6 Apart from correction of hypoglycaemia, which ONE of the following would be the most appropriate immediate first step in further management?

- [ ] A Cranial USS
- [ ] B CT scan brain
- [ ] C Liver biopsy
- [ ] D Change antibiotics
- [ ] E Repeat lumbar puncture
- [ ] F Stop enteral feeds
- [ ] G Renal biopsy
- [ ] H Start phototherapy
- [ ] I Administer sodium bicarbonate iv

25.7 What is the most likely underlying diagnosis, and which ONE investigation would you request to confirm it?

. . . .

Answers to Question 25 are on page 214

ANSWERS TO QUESTION 25

25.1 F   2 ml/kg bolus peripheral iv 10% dextrose

25.2 H   Gram-negative bacilli

25.3 H   *Escherichia coli*

25.4 B   She has a mixed hyperbilirubinaemia

       F   The low pH suggests a high acid concentration

      H   She probably has a urinary tract infection (UTI)

25.5 F   All of the above

25.6 F   Stop enteral feeds

25.7   Galactosaemia

       Assay galactose-1-phosphate uridyl transferase (G-1-P-UT)

Discussion

In a neonate with fever and vomiting a full septic screen is mandatory. In this case, lethargy, poor feeding and a full fontanelle suggest meningitis and this is confirmed on lumbar puncture. The CSF microscopy demonstrates bacilli which are pink on Gram-staining (Gram-negative) as opposed to purple blue (Gram-positive). The most likely organism is *E. coli* and its portal of entry is likely to have been the urinary tract.

Neonatal *E. coli* sepsis should always prompt consideration of galactosaemia as an underlying aetiology. Further clues in this case are persistent hypoglycaemia and acidosis, hepatomegaly with jaundice, deranged liver function and coagulopathy, and reducing substances other than glucose in the urine. The condition presents only once feeding is commenced and lactose in breast or standard formula milk is metabolised to glucose and galactose. The consequent accumulation of galactose-1-phosphate (in the absence of G-1-P-UT) is injurious to the parenchymal cells of the liver, kidney and brain. Clinistix® tests only for the presence of glucose whereas Clinitest® will detect all reducing sugars. A positive Clinitest® but negative Clinistix® therefore indicates the presence of a reducing substance other than glucose (in this case galactose).

Stopping enteral feeds and starting a galactose-free formula usually results in a dramatic improvement. However, early diagnosis by assay of galactose-1-phosphate uridyl transferase (G-1-P-UT), and dietary restriction of lactose intake do not prevent long-term complications. These include neurodevelopmental delay, (particularly in language acquisition) and premature ovarian failure in females. Endogenous production of galactose may be responsible for these long-term effects. Follow up throughout life is mandatory.

Determining the exact aetiology of hyponatraemia in the context of meningitis can be difficult as vomiting, SIADH and cerebral salt wasting (CSW), or a combination of the three, are all possible. Galactosaemia is one of the hepatorenal syndromes and patients may have a proximal renal tubulopathy. Urinary tract infection may also cause transient renal tubulopathy.

Reference

Walter, J.H., Collins, J.E., Leonard, J.V., on behalf of the UK Galactosaemia Steering Group. 1999. Recommendations for the management of galactosaemia. *Archives of Diseases in Childhood* **80**:93–96.

QUESTION 26

A 7-year-old boy is referred by his GP with a 2-day history of aching central abdominal pain. He has been reluctant to eat and drink today, and had a loose stool this morning in which some blood was seen. He has not vomited but feels sick. He denies urinary symptoms. He has developed a rash that started on his lower legs and feet and is spreading up his body. He has not complained of joint pain. Other than an upper respiratory tract infection 2 weeks ago he has been completely well recently and has not lost weight. Direct enquiry reveals no other symptoms of note.

Past medical history is otherwise unremarkable. He was born at term and was well in early infancy. He is fully immunised. There have been no concerns at school. He has a 5-year-old brother with cerebral palsy of unknown aetiology. Both parents are well and on no medication. There is no history of foreign travel.

He is afebrile and well perfused, and his heart rate is 110 beats per minute with a blood pressure of 95/60. Heart sounds are normal with no murmurs audible. Respiratory examination is normal. He is centrally tender on abdominal palpation but no masses are palpable. Bowel sounds are audible. He is alert and talking normally. Joint examination is unremarkable. He has bilateral, small, non-tender submandibular lymphadenopathy. He has a raised, non-blanching rash on his lower legs and feet.

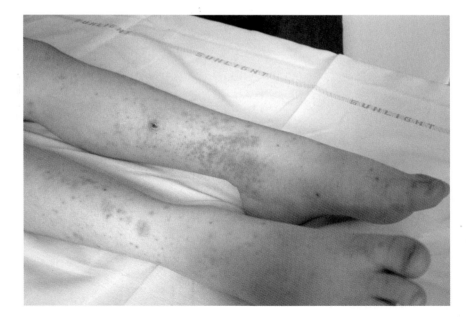

Initial investigations are as follows:

Haemoglobin:	10.2 g/dl
White cell count:	6.1×10^9/litre
Platelet count:	413×10^9/litre
Activated partial thromboplastin time:	32 seconds
Prothrombin time:	13 seconds
Fibrinogen:	3.7 g/litre
Sodium:	134 mmol/litre
Potassium:	4.7 mmol/litre
Urea:	9.9 mmol/litre
Creatinine:	47 μmol/litre
Erythrocyte sedimentation rate:	45 mm/hour
C-reactive protein:	12 g/litre
Urinalysis:	

	Leukocytes	1+
	Blood	3+
	Nitrites	–
	Protein	1+

26.1 What is the most likely clinical diagnosis?

- [ ] A Meningococcal septicaemia
- [ ] B Henoch–Schönlein purpura
- [ ] C Von Willebrand's disease
- [ ] D Rocky Mountain spotted fever
- [ ] E Erythema nodosum
- [ ] F Haemophilia A
- [ ] G Appendicitis
- [ ] H Haemophilia B
- [ ] I Acute renal failure
- [ ] J Acute promyelocytic leukaemia
- [ ] K Erythema multiforme
- [ ] L Pyoderma gangrenosum
- [ ] M Haemolytic uraemic syndrome
- [ ] N Idiopathic thrombocytopenic purpura

26.2 In addition to simple analgesia, which of the following best describes your initial management?

- [ ] A Lumbar puncture, cefotaxime, notify public health
- [ ] B Admission for close observation, prednisolone
- [ ] C Admission, stool culture, metronidazole
- [ ] D Trimethoprim 1/52, renal ultrasound, DMSA scan
- [ ] E Admission for close observation
- [ ] F More specific clotting studies
- [ ] G Immediate surgical opinion
- [ ] H Bone marrow and haematology opinion
- [ ] I Doxycycline and chloramphenicol intravenously

26.3 How do you account for the urinalysis?

- [ ] A Probable urinary tract infection
- [ ] B Secondary to nephrolithiasis
- [ ] C Bleeding from renal tumour
- [ ] D Secondary to mesangial IgA deposition
- [ ] E Probably trauma-related
- [ ] F Reflects myoglobinuria
- [ ] G As a result of disseminated intravascular coagulation
- [ ] H Haemolytic–uraemic syndrome
- [ ] I Renal vein thrombosis

Two hours after admission you are called to review him as his abdominal pain has worsened and he has passed a red mucousy stool. He has had one vomit described as green in colour. His pulse is now 120 and capillary refill time 3 seconds. He is tender to palpation in his lower abdomen, but there is no rebound or guarding. He is given a fluid bolus of 20 ml/kg and a plain abdominal X-ray is requested.

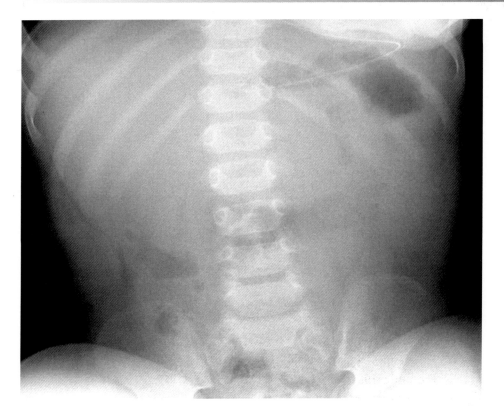

An urgent abdominal ultrasound scan is then requested.

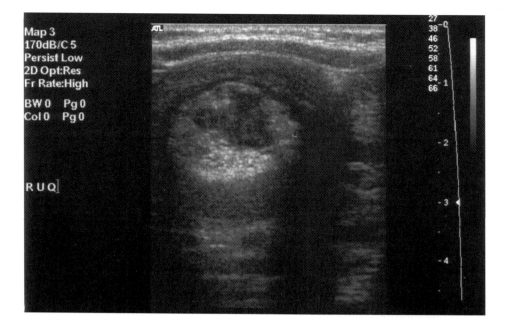

Abdominal ultrasound

26.4 What is this radiological sign called?

- [ ] A Sign de dance
- [ ] B 'Claw' sign
- [ ] C 'Apple-core' sign
- [ ] D 'Doughnut' sign
- [ ] E 'Ring' sign
- [ ] F 'String' sign

26.5   What has most likely caused his deterioration?

☐   A   Septic ileus
☐   B   Volvulus
☐   C   Intussusception
☐   D   Early tumour lysis syndrome
☐   E   Appendicitis with bowel obstruction
☐   F   Acute typhlitis
☐   G   Acute enterocolitis
☐   H   Meckel's diverticulitis

26.6   Other than a surgical opinion, which ONE definitive step in management do you think he needs next?

☐   A   Start hyperhydration and seek a haematology opinion
☐   B   Urgent laparotomy
☐   C   Intravenous antibiotic therapy
☐   D   Urgent nephrology opinion
☐   E   Technetium scintigraphy
☐   F   Mesenteric artery angiogram
☐   G   Barium swallow
☐   H   Barium enema
☐   I   Stool culture
☐   J   Air enema

Answers to Question 26 are on page 222

ANSWERS TO QUESTION 26

26.1 B   Henoch–Schönlein purpura (HSP)
26.2 E   Admission for close observation
26.3 D   Secondary to mesangial IgA deposition
26.4 D   'Doughnut' sign
26.5 C   Intussusception
26.6 J   Air enema

Discussion

HSP is an IgA-mediated small-vessel vasculitis that typically affects the skin, joints, kidneys and gastrointestinal tract. It is the most common cause of non-thrombocytopenic purpura in children, and is more common in males, winter and children aged 2–8 years. An acute onset is usual, with palpable purpura occurring in crops typically over the extensor surfaces including the buttocks. Groups of lesions tend to last 3–11 days, and may appear over intervals from a few days to a few months. There is often associated dependent oedema.

60% have renal involvement which is either present at diagnosis or develops within the first 2 months after the onset of the rash. This is limited in most to benign microscopic haematuria. A small minority develop a rapidly-progressive crescentic glomerulonephritis with acute renal failure. The condition is one of the commoner causes of renal failure in childhood.

Again, 60% have large joint arthritis usually of the knee or ankle, which is non-erosive and transient. Gut involvement is manifest by colicky abdominal pain, and more than half have diarrhoea, haematemesis or occult haem-positive stools. Intussusception may occur, as in this case, and should be suspected if there is abdominal pain and redcurrant jelly stools. An abdominal X-ray is rarely diagnostic though may show a density in the area of the intussusception, together with paucity of gas in the right lower quadrant; the diagnosis can sometimes be confirmed using ultrasound, as in this case. The classic finding is a 'loop within a loop' of bowel, termed the 'doughnut' sign (see figure opposite).

Reduction is usually achieved by air enema, though if this fails or there is a suspicion of perforation surgical reduction is mandatory.

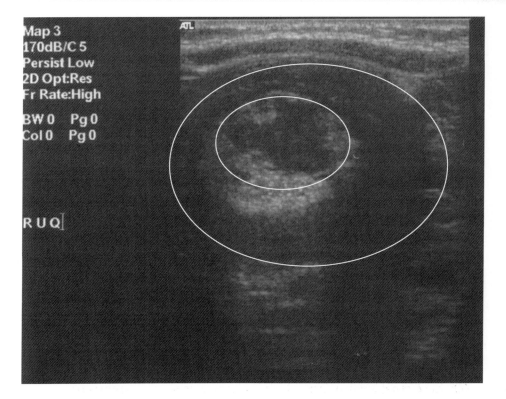

Other reported rare complications include orchitis, a CNS vasculitis manifest by seizures, hemiparesis and coma, and hepatosplenomegaly, pancreatitis and mononeuritis.

Treatment is largely symptomatic with simple analgesia and rest. Management of renal involvement is the same as for other forms of glomerulonephritis. Surgical treatment is required for bowel perforation and testicular torsion, and for intussusception not correctable with air enema. Corticosteroids (1–2 mg/kg per day) are rarely used and largely reserved for those with CNS or severe gastrointestinal involvement. The overall prognosis is excellent, although 1 in 50–100 suffer long-term renal morbidity. Long-term follow-up is mandatory (annual blood pressure and urinalysis) as chronic renal failure is a well-reported complication (1%) and may develop as long as 15 years after the original presentation.

In this case, none of the other suggested diagnoses in Question 26.1 are likely. The raised non-blanching nature of the rash in this clinical context suggests it to be 'palpable purpura', classical of HSP. The purpura in meningococcal septicaemia is usually non-palpable and accompanied by some evidence of disseminated intravascular coagulation in a febrile child. Haemophilia usually presents with easy bruising, intramuscular haematomas and haemarthroses and a prolonged APTT. Von Willebrand's disease is typically manifest by mucocutaneous haemorrhage, including excessive bruising, epistaxis and menorrhagia, sometimes accompanied by a prolonged APTT. Erythema nodosum is a paniculitis usually confined to the pretibial area. Appendicitis does not usually present with gastrointestinal haemorrhage. From the information provided there is insufficient evidence to support a diagnosis of acute renal failure or acute promyelocytic leukaemia. The nature of the rash and its distribution are quite unlike either erythema multiforme or pyoderma gangrenosum.

QUESTION 27

You are asked to review a baby boy who is now 4 hours old. On the day of delivery his mother attended the delivery suite in established labour. In discussion with the attending obstetrician it transpires that the delivery was expedited by EMLSCS because of fetal bradycardia. The CTG was otherwise normal. Cord gases were pH 7.37 (arterial) and 7.34 (venous). He was born in good condition and, although the neonatal team were at the delivery, no resuscitation was required and he was quickly handed back to his parents. The pregnancy has been otherwise straightforward. Mother's booking serology was unremarkable. She was well during her pregnancy with no specific problems and no concern regarding fetal movements. An anomaly scan was normal at 21 week's gestation. There is no family history of note except that a second cousin had an atrial septal defect which was repaired at 8 years of age.

He is now 4 hours old and you have been called back to the postnatal ward because the midwifery team are concerned that his heart rate is slow and irregular. He has had a 12-lead ECG which shows a normal QRS axis and no evidence of ventricular hypertrophy. A short rhythm strip is available for your perusal.

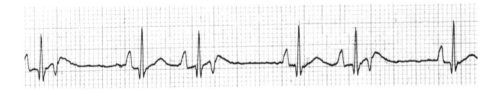

He is initially asleep when you start examining him. He is not dysmorphic. Cardiac output is clinically good and he is pink. Right arm mean blood pressure is 42 mmHg. Peripheral pulses are normal. Heart rate is variable and you estimate it to be initially 85 beats per minute, quickening to a more regular 140 beats per minute when he wakes up. The rhythm sounds irregular. Heart sounds are normal with a grade 1/6 soft systolic murmur loudest beneath the left clavicle. The work of breathing is normal and breath sounds are vesicular. The liver is just palpable beneath the right costal margin. The remainder of the first day check is normal.

27.1   What does this rhythm strip show?

☐ A   Complete heart block
☐ B   Sinus arrhythmia
☐ C   First-degree heart block
☐ D   Blocked atrial ectopic beats
☐ E   Second-degree heart block (Mobitz type I)
☐ F   Second-degree heart block (Mobitz type II)
☐ G   Normal rhythm
☐ H   Biphasic T waves
☐ I   Prolonged QT_c interval

27.2   Which investigation would you request next?

☐ A   No further investigation is required
☐ B   Echocardiogram
☐ C   Neonatal anti-Ro antibody
☐ D   Maternal anti-Ro antibody
☐ E   24-hour ECG
☐ F   Maternal anti double-stranded DNA antibody
☐ G   Maternal anti nuclear antibody
☐ H   Neonatal full blood count

27.3   What is the most likely unifying diagnosis?

☐ A   Corrected transposition of the great arteries
☐ B   Ventricular septal defect
☐ C   Maternal systemic lupus erythematosus
☐ D   Atrial septal defect
☐ E   Pulmonary stenosis
☐ F   There is no specific unifying diagnosis
☐ G   Wolff–Parkinson–White syndrome
☐ H   Ebstein's anomaly
☐ I   Congenital long QT syndrome

Answers to Question 27 are on page 228

ANSWERS TO QUESTION 27

27.1 D   Blocked atrial ectopic beats
27.2 A   No further investigation is required
27.3 F   There is no specific unifying diagnosis

Discussion

This is a relatively common clinical finding in the newborn period. Delivery was expedited in the face of an apparent fetal bradycardia, which was interpreted as a potential marker of fetal distress. However, the CTG was otherwise normal and this baby was born in good condition and had normal cord gases. There is no history to suggest maternal lupus (which may cause congenital heart block) or a long QT syndrome, and the normal anomaly scan at 21 weeks' gestation makes the diagnoses of either Ebstein's anomaly or (severe) pulmonary stenosis unlikely. The history of a cousin requiring surgery for an ASD does not increase this baby's risk of having congenital heart disease as only such a history in a first-degree relative would be relevant.

   The key history when this baby is reviewed at 4 hours of age is that the heart rate, though variable when asleep, is still within the normal range for a sleeping term baby. It quickens on wakening (sympathetic drive) to a more regular rate. This normal physiological phenomenon together with the rhythm strip provided exclude the other differential diagnoses listed. The presence of a 'P' with every 'QRS' excludes complete heart block. The constant PR interval of 0.16 s excludes both first- (abnormally long PR interval) and second-degree heart block (Mobitz types I and II). The corrected QT interval ($QT_c = QT/\sqrt{RR}$) of 0.35 s is well within the normal range (0–6 months < 0.49 s, > 6 months 0.425 s). Sinus arrhythmia could result in a similar sounding clinical presentation, but it is the presence of a number of premature atrial contractions (PAC) occurring on the 'T' wave (when the ventricle is repolarising and therefore refractory to conduction) that seals the diagnosis in this case.

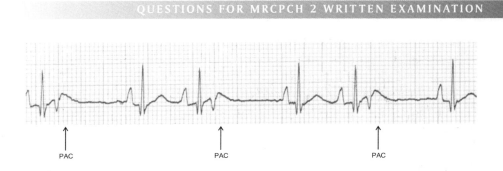

This phenomenon typically vanishes by 3 months of age, though is associated with an increased risk of supraventricular tachycardia during this time. No further investigation is required in the neonatal period in an otherwise well baby, and no specific follow up is necessary beyond early infancy.

QUESTION 28

You are called to review a 12-day-old premature infant who has deteriorated over the evening. In brief, he was born by emergency caesarean section for maternal abruption at 27+5 weeks' gestation. He was small for dates with a birthweight of 700 g. Cord gases were: arterial pH 7.1, venous pH 6.9. He was successfully resuscitated, given surfactant, ventilated and transferred to the NICU. There were no perinatal risk factors for sepsis.

Progress over the first 12 days of life has been fairly good. Initial hyaline membrane disease was moderate and he was extubated successfully to nasal CPAP on day 5. However, he developed a progressive uncompensated hypercapnia and was reventilated on day 7. Current ventilation is SIMV p(16/4) RR30 and he has been in air for the last 48 hours. He is fluid restricted to 120 ml/kg per day for a PDA diagnosed clinically on day 10. He was started on 1 ml/hour of EBM as trophic enteral feeds via nasogastric tube on day 9, and these have been liberalised over the last 24 hours, increasing by 1 ml every 4–6 hours. The neonatal nurses report that over the last 24 hours he has become very sicky and uncomfortable. Vomiting is non-bilious. He has just passed a large dark liquid stool and has a mildly distended abdomen.

On examination he is afebrile with a heart rate of 170, BP 60/20 and respiratory rate of 60. His ventilation settings have not been changed but he has developed an oxygen requirement. He has good chest expansion bilaterally. On auscultation there is no audible murmur. Peripheral pulses are prominent. Abdominal palpation is clearly painful and there are visible loops of bowel. Bowel sounds are present. His umbilicus looks moist but there is no periumbilical flare. Examination is otherwise unremarkable.

Initial blood results are as follows:

Haemoglobin:	12.0 g/dl
White cell count:	2.4×10^9/litre
Platelets:	73×10^9/litre
Sodium	130 mmol/l
Potassium	4.0 mmol/l
Urea	4 mmol/l
Creat	35 μmol/l

Arterial blood gas

pH	7.25
pO_2	6.4 kPa
pCO_2	5.0 kPa
HCO_3^-	15 mmol/l
BE	−10
FiO_2	0.35

LFT and coagulation screen   Unremarkable.

Abdominal x-ray:
Dilated loops of bowel, with air visible as far as the rectum

28.1   What is the most likely diagnosis?

- [ ] A   Sepsis
- [ ] B   Gastroenteritis
- [ ] C   GORD
- [ ] D   Tracheo-oesophageal fistula
- [ ] E   Oesophageal web
- [ ] F   Duodenal atresia
- [ ] G   Malrotation
- [ ] H   Necrotising enterocolitis
- [ ] I   Hirschsprung's disease
- [ ] J   Meconium ileus
- [ ] K   Meconium plug syndrome
- [ ] L   Anal atresia
- [ ] M   UTI

28.2   What is your immediate management?

- [ ] A   Stop enteral feeds and rechallenge in 4 hours starting at 1 ml/h
- [ ] B   Commence trial of ranitidine for suspected gastro-oesophageal reflux disease
- [ ] C   Fluid resuscitation; full septic screen; commence ceftriaxone and gentamicin. Fluid restrict to 100 ml/kg per day
- [ ] D   Fluid resuscitation; blood culture, urine culture; commence ceftriaxone and gentamicin. Fluid restrict to 100 ml/kg per day
- [ ] E   Fluid resuscitation; full septic screen; commence ceftriaxone and gentamicin. Commence indomethacin

☐ F Fluid resuscitation; blood culture, urine culture; commence ceftriaxone and gentamicin. Commence indomethacin

☐ G Fluid resuscitation; full septic screen; stop enteral feeds; commence ceftriaxone, gentamicin and metronidazole

☐ H Fluid resuscitation; blood culture, urine culture, stop enteral feeds; commence ceftriaxone, gentamicin and metronidazole

☐ I Fluid resuscitation; full septic screen; stop enteral feeds; commence ceftriaxone, gentamicin and metronidazole. Fluid restrict to 100 ml/kg per day

☐ J Fluid resuscitation; blood cultures, urine culture, stop enteral feeds; commence ceftriaxone, gentamicin and metronidazole. Fluid restrict to 100 ml/kg per day

☐ K Fluid resuscitation; full septic screen; stop enteral feeds; commence ceftriaxone, gentamicin and metronidazole. Commence indomethacin

☐ L Fluid resuscitation; blood cultures, urine culture, stop enteral feeds; commence ceftriaxone, gentamicin and metronidazole. Commence indomethacin

28.3 Which FOUR predisposing factors does this infant have for this clinical scenario?

☐ A Evidence of periumbilical infection
☐ B IUGR
☐ C Male sex
☐ D Patent ductus arteriosus
☐ E Evidence of prolonged perinatal hypoxia
☐ F Hypertonic formula feeds
☐ G Umbilical catheterisation
☐ H Polycythaemia
☐ I History of exchange transfusion
☐ J Overventilation
☐ K Permissive hypercapnia
☐ L Prolonged chest disease
☐ M History of failed extubation
☐ N Prematurity

Overnight, his abdomen becomes more distended. He develops bilious NG aspirates but his vomiting has stopped. On examination his abdomen is tense, distended and intensely painful despite opiate analgesia. He has not passed further stools.

28.4   What would best explain his current predicament?

. . . .

28.5   Which ONE test from the list below would you perform to confirm the diagnosis?

☐   A   Cranial ultrasound
☐   B   Chest X-ray
☐   C   AP abdominal X-ray
☐   D   Cross-table lateral abdominal X-ray
☐   E   Abdominal ultrasound
☐   F   Air enema
☐   G   CT chest
☐   H   CT abdomen
☐   I   MIBG scan

Answers to Question 28 are on page 234

ANSWERS TO QUESTION 28

28.1 H Necrotising enterocolitis

28.2 J Fluid resuscitation; blood cultures, urine culture, stop enteral feeds; commence ceftriaxone, gentamicin and metronidazole. Fluid restrict to 100 ml/kg per day

28.3 B IUGR

D Patent ductus arteriosus

E Evidence of prolonged perinatal hypoxia

N Prematurity

28.4 Gastrointestinal perforation secondary to necrotising enterocolitis

28.5 D Cross-table lateral abdominal X-ray

Discussion

Establishing enteral feeds in premature infants is often problematic as bowel motility is only fully functional by 36 weeks in utero. Consequently, large aspirates, vomiting, unpredictable bowel movements and bowel distension may all occur around the time when enteral feeding is being established. As a result, early signs of NEC may be overlooked. Cardinal signs of NEC include bilious vomiting, abdominal distension, severe pain, bloody diarrhoea, metabolic acidosis and shock. Thrombocytopenia occurs early in the disease and may be the first sign of an unhealthy bowel. Neutropenia is common. Hyponatraemia, hypovolaemia and acidosis occur secondary to fluid collection in the gut.

The abdominal film may be normal early in the illness. Radiological findings pertinent to NEC are bowel distension, bowel wall thickening, pneumatosis intestinalis and transient gas in the portal veins. Perforation is a serious complication which must be suspected with any deterioration, and is best confirmed with a cross-table lateral abdominal X-ray or lateral decubitus X-ray. Free air is commonly seen beneath the umbilicus but may also be visualised in pockets outlining the falciform ligament or in the hepatorenal space on a lateral decubitus X-ray.

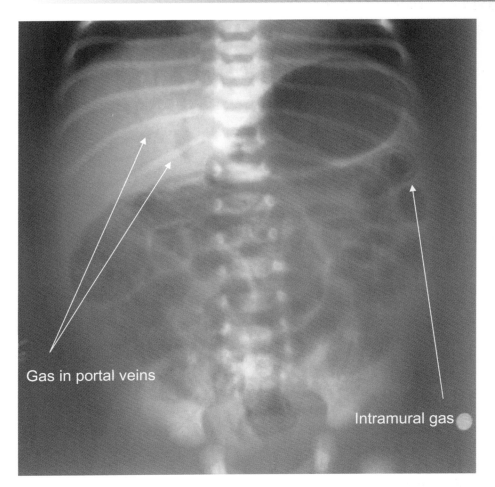

Gas in portal veins

Intramural gas

Abdominal x-ray showing pneumatosis intestinalis and visible gas in the portal veins

The aetiology of NEC is not fully understood but there are three main predisposing factors:

- mucosal injury
- infection
- feeding.

Mucosal injury may occur as a consequence of cellular hypoxia from prolonged hypoxia at birth, or from decreased gut perfusion either in utero as a result of reversed end diastolic flow (associated with IUGR), or postnatally with polycythaemia, umbilical artery catheterisation, exchange

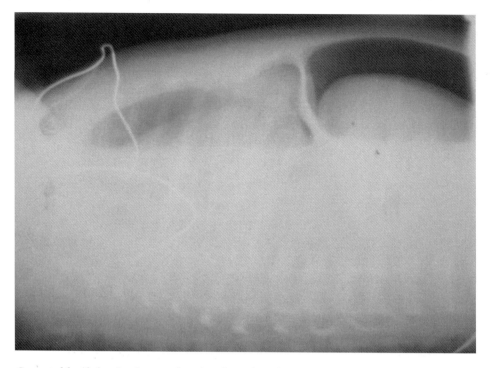

Cross-table abdominal x-ray showing bowel perforation

transfusion, ductal steal from a PDA or indomethacin. Direct injury from hyperosmolar feeds and bacterial pathogens may also precipitate NEC.

The red cell T-antigen (Thomsen–Friedenreich cryptantigen or TCA) is a naturally occurring concealed red cell antigen, which is exposed by neuraminidases produced by many bacteria. Although no single pathogen has been defined as causative in NEC, many infants with NEC have T-antigen activation and are susceptible to anti-T-antigen antibody-mediated haemolysis. These infants should receive T-antigen antibody-negative blood should they require blood transfusion.

Infants with NEC without perforation are best treated conservatively with triple antibiotic therapy and exclusion of enteral feeds for at least 10 days. Indications for surgical intervention with resection of necrotic bowel include perforation and progression of disease despite optimal medical management.

Complications of NEC include stricture formation, short bowel syndrome from bowel resection, recurrence and protracted lactose intolerance.

QUESTION 29

You are asked to see a 13-month-old boy in A&E with fever, rash and a swollen face. He is an otherwise well child, born at term with no perinatal complications. He was admitted to hospital at 3 months of age with RSV bronchiolitis requiring oxygen therapy and orogastric feeding and has been a chesty baby since. He has been treated for otitis media on one occasion by his GP. His growth and development have been normal and he has received all his vaccinations. He is an only child. The family have not been abroad. They spent their summer holiday in the New Forest.

Mother reports that he has been unwell for 4 or 5 days with high fever, poor feeding and lethargy. He developed spots 3 days ago, which mother thought looked like chicken pox and these have continued to develop. Some lesions have crusted. She is more worried now because over the afternoon he has become more feverish and lethargic and isn't responding to her as normal. He has passed green liquid stool.

On examination his temperature 40.5°C, pulse 170, blood pressure 100/50, respiratory rate 50 and oxygen saturation 97% in air. He is lethargic and miserable and looks uniformly flushed. Perfusion is good with capillary refill time of 1 second. He has bilateral injected non-suppurative conjunctivae. He has a few skin lesions scattered over all limbs, his trunk and scalp. He has a quiet systolic murmur. His chest sounds clear and his abdomen is soft with no visceromegaly. ENT examination is unremarkable. He has shotty cervical lymphadenopathy. Urinalysis reveals leukocytes +, protein + + +, blood +, nitrite –, SG 1030.

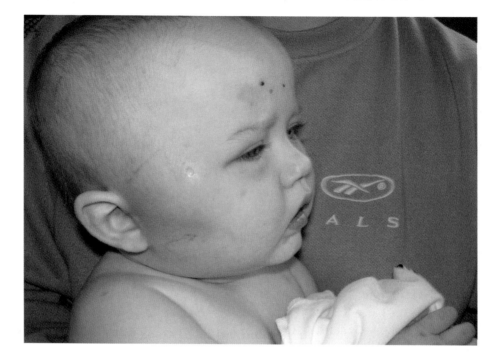

29.1 Which THREE diagnoses collectively describe this child's predicament?

- ☐ A Chicken pox
- ☐ B Meningococcal septicaemia
- ☐ C Meningococcal meningitis
- ☐ D Lyme disease
- ☐ E Post-septal periorbital cellulitis
- ☐ F Pre-septal periorbital cellulitis
- ☐ G Right-sided facial subcutaneous abscess
- ☐ H Weil's disease
- ☐ I Pneumococcal septicaemia
- ☐ J Toxic shock syndrome
- ☐ K Urinary tract infection
- ☐ L Stevens–Johnson syndrome
- ☐ M Erythema multiforme
- ☐ N Kawasaki disease
- ☐ O Subacute infective endocarditis
- ☐ P Measles

29.2 Which EIGHT interventions would you undertake at this stage?

☐ A CT scan brain including sinus cuts
☐ B Blood culture, blood count, renal and liver function, inflammatory markers
☐ C Clotting profile including fibrinogen
☐ D Venous blood gas
☐ E Group and save blood, request availability of fresh frozen plasma
☐ F Immune profile
☐ G Chest X-ray
☐ H Lumbar puncture
☐ I Throat swab
☐ J Oral antibiotics
☐ K Benzyl penicillin and flucloxacillin iv
☐ L Cefotaxime and clindamycin iv
☐ M 20 ml/kg volume resuscitation, with review and one repeat bolus if needed
☐ N Transfer to paediatric ward
☐ O Transfer to paediatric HDU
☐ P Transfer to regional PICU
☐ Q Inform anaesthetist of need for potential early intubation

A venous blood gas is taken:

pH:	7.28
pO_2:	5.0 kPa
pCO_2	5.0 kPa
HCO_3^-:	17 mmol/litre
BE:	−8

29.3 Interpret the initial venous blood gas above

☐ A Metabolic acidosis with respiratory alkalosis
☐ B Metabolic acidosis with respiratory alkalosis and hypoxia
☐ C Metabolic acidosis
☐ D Respiratory acidosis
☐ E Mixed metabolic and respiratory acidosis
☐ F Normal gas

After 40 ml/kg volume resuscitation, you review him while still in A&E. Observations are P 160, BP 95/30, RR 60, oxygen saturation 92% in air. He is more lethargic.
   Blood results are as follows:

Haemoglobin:	13.4 g/dl
White cell count:	20.9×10^9/litre
Platelets:	71×10^9/litre
PT:	23 seconds
APTT:	65 seconds
Fibrinogen:	1.2 g/litre
Na:	129 mmol/litre
K:	4.1 mmol/litre
Urea:	23 mmol/litre
Creatinine:	174 μmol/litre
iCa:	0.66 mmol/litre
Mg:	0.55 mmol/litre
ALT:	55 IU/litre
Bilirubin:	25 μmol/litre
Glucose:	10.2 mmol/litre
pH:	7.25
pO_2:	4.5 kPa
pCO_2:	3.2 kPa
HCO_3^-:	17 mmol/litre
BE:	−8

29.4   Interpret the venous blood gas above

- [ ] A   Metabolic acidosis with compensatory respiratory alkalosis
- [ ] B   Metabolic acidosis with compensatory respiratory alkalosis and hypoxia
- [ ] C   Metabolic acidosis
- [ ] D   Respiratory acidosis
- [ ] E   Mixed metabolic and respiratory acidosis
- [ ] F   Normal gas

29.5 What are the FOUR most important further interventions at this stage?

☐ A Lumbar puncture
☐ B CT brain
☐ C Emergency sinus surgery
☐ D Further aggressive fluid resuscitation with normal saline
☐ E Further aggressive fluid resuscitation with 20% human albumin solution
☐ F Calcium correction iv
☐ G Magnesium correction iv
☐ H 20 ml/kg fresh frozen plasma
☐ I 10 ml/kg whole blood
☐ J 10 ml/kg platelets
☐ K Immediate intubation and ventilation by anaesthetist
☐ L Urinary catheterisation
☐ M Commence inotropic support

Answers to Question 29 are on page 242

ANSWERS TO QUESTION 29

29.1 A Chicken pox
     G Right-sided facial subcutaneous abscess
     J Toxic shock syndrome
29.2 B Blood culture, blood count, renal and liver function, inflammatory
       markers
     C Clotting profile including fibrinogen
     D Venous blood gas
     E Group and save blood, request availability of fresh frozen plasma
     L Cefotaxime and clindamycin iv
     M 20 ml/kg volume resuscitation, with review and one repeat bolus if
       needed
     O Transfer to paediatric HDU
     Q Inform anaesthetist of need for potential early intubation
29.3 C Metabolic acidosis
29.4 A Metabolic acidosis with compensatory respiratory alkalosis
29.5 D Further aggressive fluid resuscitation with normal saline
     H 20 ml/kg fresh frozen plasma
     K Immediate intubation and ventilation by anaesthetist
     M Commence inotropic support

Discussion

Staphylococcal toxic shock syndrome is a severe multisystem disease characterized by hypotension, fever, a diffuse erythematous rash that desquamates and multi-organ failure secondary to capillary leak and shock.

Staphylococcal toxic shock syndrome is a superantigen-mediated disease. In the majority of cases in children the focus of infection is a cutaneous or subcutaneous infection, and primary varicella with staphylococcal superinfection is a typical example. The staphylococcal infection itself may be trivial in comparison with the severity of the toxin-mediated pathology. The toxin responsible is the **superantigen TSST** (staph enterotoxin F).

Superantigens have been shown to be responsible for staphylococcal and streptococcal toxic shock syndromes. They have been implicated in many other illnesses including:

- Scalded skin syndrome
- Scarlet fever
- Kawasaki's disease
- Autoimmune diseases.

Specific diagnostic criteria

- Fever > 38.9°C
- Rash:Diffuse, erythematous
  - With desquamation 1–2 weeks after onset of illness
- Hypotension/shock
- Involvement of three or more of following organ systems
  - Mucous membranes: vaginal, conjunctival, oropharyngeal hyperaemia
  - Gastrointestinal: vomiting, profuse diarrhoea
  - Muscular: severe myalgia, raised CK
  - Renal: raised urea/creatinine
  - Hepatic: hepatitis
  - Haematology: thrombocytopenia
  - CNS: disorientation/altered consciousness
- Exclusion of Rocky Mountain spotted fever/leptospirosis/measles

---

QUESTION 30

Consider each of the following conditions:

List A

A   Ethylene glycol ingestion
B   Diabetes mellitus
C   Salicylate ingestion
D   Methylmalonic acidaemia
E   Propionyl CoA carboxylase deficiency
F   Acute renal failure
G   Adrenal disorder
H   Acetazolamide therapy
I   Septicaemia
J   Severe diarrhoea
K   Acute subdural haematoma
L   Methanol ingestion
M   Iron poisoning
N   Alcohol ingestion
O   Viral encephalitis
P   Distal renal tubular acidosis (type I)
Q   Metformin ingestion

Consider each of the following case histories:

Case I

History

A 4-year-old boy is brought to casualty by his parents at 10 pm concerned that he is drowsy. They are part of a large travelling family. He has been in the care of their two daughters, aged 16 and 14, all afternoon. The girls say he has been vomiting, has complained of 'tummy ache and funny eyes', and has been sleepy. He opened his bowels normally that morning. The girls say that they spent the morning on the campsite playing ball games, and then cooked some lunch on the stove before going out for a walk. They don't think he has had an accident. He has never previously been in hospital and is not immunised. Mother is a non-insulin dependent diabetic and is on some tablets that she can't remember the name of. Father is well, though smells of alcohol. The remainder of the immediate family are well. They are not known to the local social services.

Examination

Temperature is 36.7°C, heart rate 100, blood pressure 88/57 and respiratory rate 26. Heart sounds are normal with no murmurs. There is good air entry bilaterally with no added sounds. He groans on deep palpation of the upper abdomen. There is no organomegaly and bowel sounds are audible. Glasgow Coma Scale score is 11. Pupils are 7mm bilaterally, non-reactive to light. There are no gross abnormalities of the peripheral nervous system. Reflexes are normal with flexor plantars.

Initial investigations

Haemoglobin:	12.2 g/dl
White cell count:	7.3×10^9/litre
Platelets:	449×10^9/litre
ESR:	8 mm/hour
Sodium:	134 mmol/litre
Potassium:	4.0 mmol/litre
Urea:	5.9 mmol/litre
Creatinine:	55 μmol/litre
Glucose:	6.8 mmol/litre
Venous pH:	7.17
Bicarbonate:	13 mmol/litre
Serum osmolality:	322 mosm/kg
Chloride:	102 mmol/litre
Ammonia:	52 μmol/litre
Lactate:	2.2 mmol/litre
$paCO_2$:	5.7 kPa

30.1 **Which ONE of the following clinical descriptions correspond to a Glasgow Coma Scale score (GCS) of 11?**

- [ ] A Eye opening to voice, consolable crying, localises pain
- [ ] B Eye opening to pain, persistently irritable, withdraws to pain
- [ ] C Eye opening to voice, persistently irritable, localises pain
- [ ] D Eye opening to pain, restless and agitated, extends to pain
- [ ] E Spontaneous eye opening, consolable crying, localises pain
- [ ] F Eye opening to voice, persistently irritable, withdraws to pain
- [ ] G Eye opening to pain, restless and agitated, flexes to pain
- [ ] H Spontaneous eye opening, consolable crying, obeys commands
- [ ] I Eye opening to pain, persistently irritable, flexes to pain

30.2   What is the anion gap?

- [ ] A   25
- [ ] B   8
- [ ] C   −25
- [ ] D   20
- [ ] E   19
- [ ] F   23
- [ ] G   6
- [ ] H   10

30.3   Which of the diagnoses in list A above is most likely?

. . . .

30.4   Which ONE of the following is most likely to help you secure
       the diagnosis?

- [ ] A   Blood culture
- [ ] B   Urine Clinistix®
- [ ] C   Blood ethanol level
- [ ] D   CT scan brain
- [ ] E   Stool culture
- [ ] F   Blood salicylate level
- [ ] G   Calculated osmolality
- [ ] H   Urine organic acids
- [ ] I   Urine steroid profile
- [ ] J   Blood iron level
- [ ] K   CSF viral culture/PCR HSV
- [ ] L   MRI scan brain
- [ ] M   Synacthen test
- [ ] N   HbA1c

Case 2

History

*At 8 am a 14-year-old girl is brought to casualty by her parents having been found
walking around the garden 4 hours previously. When asked, she could not remember
getting out of bed. Her parents have become concerned because she is now difficult*

to rouse. She had complained of a frontal headache and had vomited once the day before, and had been given 500 mg paracetamol before going to bed. Whilst being seen, she wets herself and then has a 2-minute right-sided focal seizure.

Examination (post-ictal)

Temperature is 38.7°C, heart rate 100, blood pressure 125/60 and respiratory rate 10. Heart sounds are normal with no murmurs. Air entry is quiet bilaterally with no added sounds. Her abdomen is non-tender. There is no organomegaly. Bowel sounds are audible. Glasgow Coma Scale score is 7. Gag reflex is present. Pupils are 4 mm bilaterally, reactive to light. There is no asymmetry in limb tone. Reflexes are: arms normal; knee and ankle jerks normal; plantars: right extensor, left flexor.

Initial investigations

Haemoglobin:	13.1g/dl
White cell count:	9.3×10^9/litre
Platelets:	344×10^9/litre
ESR:	17 mm/hour
Sodium:	130 mmol/litre
Potassium:	4.7 mmol/litre
Urea:	2.1 mmol/litre
Creatinine:	59 μmol/litre
Glucose:	8.9 mmol/litre
Venous pH:	7.25
Bicarbonate:	19 mmol/litre
Serum osmolality:	292 mosm/kg
Chloride:	105 mmol/litre
Ammonia:	45 μmol/litre
Lactate:	1.9 mmol/litre
$paCO_2$:	7.7 kPa

30.5   Which of the diagnoses in List A is most likely?

. . . .

30.6   Which ONE of the following is the most important immediate investigation to carry out next?

- [ ] A   Blood culture
- [ ] B   Urine Clinistix®
- [ ] C   Blood ethanol level
- [ ] D   CT scan brain
- [ ] E   Stool culture
- [ ] F   Blood salicylate level
- [ ] G   Calculated osmolality
- [ ] H   Urine organic acids
- [ ] I   Urine steroid profile
- [ ] J   Blood iron level
- [ ] K   CSF viral culture/PCR HSV
- [ ] L   MRI scan brain
- [ ] M   Synacthen test
- [ ] N   Pregnancy test

Case 3

History

A 15-year-old known diabetic girl presents to casualty having collapsed at school. She has had a heavy cold for the last 3 days and says she hasn't had much of an appetite all week. Although her sugars have tended to be on the low side for the last 2 weeks, she has continued to administer her insulin as per normal. Her last dose was given 6 hours ago. Her parents say she has been in trouble at school because in recent weeks she has refused to participate in the physical education class, saying she feels 'tired'. Before going to school this morning she complained of abdominal pain. Once at school she tried playing tennis but complained of feeling weak, vomited twice and then fainted.

Examination

Temperature is 35.8°C, heart rate 125, blood pressure 125/55, respiratory rate 24. Heart sounds are normal with no murmurs. There is good air entry bilaterally with no added sounds. Abdomen is tender centrally, with no rebound, guarding or organomegaly; bowel sounds are audible. Glasgow Coma Scale score is 15. Cranial nerves and peripheral nervous system examination is normal.

Initial investigations

Haemoglobin:	11.1 g/dl
White cell count:	8.9×10^9/litre
Neutrophils:	4.4×10^9/litre
Lymphocytes:	1.5×10^9/litre
Monocytes:	0.6×10^9/litre
Eosinophils:	2.4×10^9/litre
Platelets:	344×10^9/litre
ESR:	17 mm/hour
Glucose:	2.1 mmol/litre
Venous pH:	7.24
Bicarbonate:	17 mmol/litre
Serum osmolality:	262 mosm/kg
Urine:	ketones 2+, sodium 85 mmol/litre
Sodium:	123 mmol/litre
Potassium:	6.8 mmol/litre
Urea:	6.1 mmol/litre
Creatinine:	59 μmol/litre
Chloride:	92 mmol/litre
Ammonia:	34 μmol/litre
Lactate:	1.5 mmol/litre
$paCO_2$:	4.7kPa

30.7   Which of the diagnoses in List A is most likely?

. . . .

30.8 After appropriate emergency treatment, which ONE of the following is most likely to help you secure the diagnosis?

☐ A Blood culture
☐ B Haemoglobin A1c
☐ C Blood ethanol level
☐ D CT scan brain
☐ E Stool culture
☐ F Blood salicylate level
☐ G Calculated osmolality
☐ H Urine organic acids
☐ I Urine steroid profile
☐ J Blood iron level
☐ K CSF viral culture/PCR HSV
☐ L MRI scan brain
☐ M Synacthen test

Answers to Question 30 are on page 252

ANSWERS TO QUESTION 30

30.1 C Eye opening to voice, persistently irritable, localises pain
30.2 E 19
30.3 L Methanol ingestion
30.4 G Calculated osmolality
30.5 O Viral encephalitis
30.6 D CT brain scan
30.7 G Adrenal disorder
30.8 M Synacthen test

Discussion

When faced with a child with acidaemia, history and physical examination and a few simple investigations (figure on p. 255) will usually point towards the underlying diagnosis.

The anion gap reflects unmeasured anions which in combination with chloride and bicarbonate counterbalance the positive charge of sodium ions:

$$\text{Anion gap} = Na^+ + (Cl^- + HCO_3^-)$$

The normal anion gap is 12 mmol/l, range 8–16 mmol/l. Elevation of the gap occurs secondary to an excessive accumulation of acids (ingested or endogenous) or as a result of inadequate excretion of acids. The anion gap may be falsely lowered in the presence of hypoalbuminaemia, hypercalcaemia and hypokalaemia. Hyperchloraemia is a typical finding in metabolic acidosis with a normal anion gap. An elevated anion gap (such as in Case 1) should prompt calculation of the osmolal gap (measured osmolality – calculated osmolality), the difference between the measured and calculated osmolality. The normal maximum difference is 15 mmol/litre. A difference greater than this suggests unmeasured osmotic particles, which in the case of toxic ingestion points towards either methanol or ethylene glycol.

Features of methanol intoxication include obtundation, severe abdominal pain, dizziness, severe metabolic acidosis, blurred vision leading to blindness, and eventual coma with respiratory depression. This differs slightly from that of ethylene glycol ingestion, which usually causes early ataxia, dysarthria, and nystagmus followed by convulsions, coma and cardiorespiratory collapse within 24 hours of ingestion. Acute tubular necrosis can develop later. Management in both cases should be in an appropriate centre in close liaison with the regional poisons unit.

Case 2 describes a girl with a recent onset of odd behaviour and headache who has become drowsy, was incontinent of urine and then had a focal seizure. On examination she is febrile, comatose and hypoventilating. Her blood results indicate she has a respiratory acidosis. Although the presentation suggests she has an encephalitis, intubation and ventilation with a prompt CT scan brain is mandatory to exclude a space-occupying lesion or other cause of raised intracranial pressure. Once the latter have been excluded CSF can then safely be obtained to confirm or refute the provisional diagnosis of encephalitis.

Case 3 describes a girl with known diabetes who on the surface one might initially think has presented in DKA. However, the history of malaise and low energy levels stretching back over a few weeks should raise the spectre of an alternative diagnosis, in this instance Addison's disease. Though rare, this condition is more common in children with diabetes mellitus. The clues in the investigations are the hypoglycaemia (not typical of DKA), hyponatraemia, hyperkalaemia, the normal anion gap (14 mmol/litre), metabolic acidosis and the high urinary sodium losses. Eosinophilia may also be present. Ketonuria is not an uncommon finding in this condition and is not exclusive to DKA in the context of an unwell child with diabetes.

The Glasgow Coma Scale is a quantitative measure of level of consciousness, and has been modified from its original form to make it more applicable to children:

Score	Eye opening
4	Spontaneous
3	To speech
2	To pain
1	None

Score	Best 'verbal' response		
	Adult/adolescent	Child	Young child
5	Oriented	Appropriate	Smiles, fixes and follows
4	Confused	Inappropriate	Cries but consolable
3	Inappropriate	Moaning	Inconsolable, irritable
2	Incomprehensible	Restless and agitated	
1		None	

Score	Best motor response
6	Follows commands or spontaneous appropriate movement
5	Localises pain
4	Withdraws to pain
3	Decorticate (flexor) posturing
2	Decerebrate (extensor) posturing
1	None

References

Barceloux, D.G., Bond, G.R., Krenzelok, E.P., Cooper, H., Vale, J.A. 2002. American Academy of Clinical Toxicology Ad Hoc Committee on the Treatment Guidelines for Methanol Poisoning. American Academy of Clinical Toxicology practice guidelines on the treatment of methanol poisoning. *Journal of Toxicology and Clinical Toxicology* **40**:415–46.

National Poisons Information Service. – **www.spib.axl.co.uk**

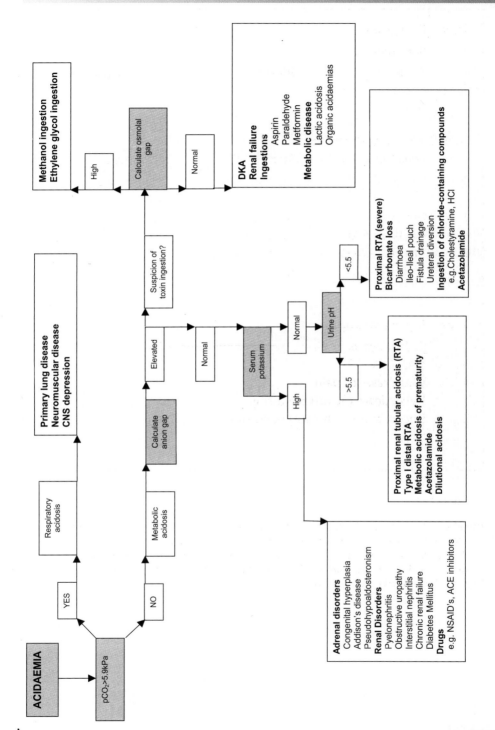

QUESTION 31

This question is about patterns of growth in the first 3 years of life. The following are a list of causes of abnormal growth during this period:

I   Undernutrition

II   Constitutional growth delay

III   Central nervous system abnormalities

IV   Genetic short stature

V   Endocrinopathies

VI   Chromosomal aberrations

VII Skeletal dysplasia

VIII In utero and perinatal insults

Three growth charts are illustrated. For each growth chart, indicate which group of diagnoses would most commonly follow the pattern of growth illustrated.

Chart One	*Chart Two*	*Chart Three*
☐ A I	☐ A I	☐ A I
☐ B II, IV, V, VII	☐ B III, V, VII	☐ B III, V, VII
☐ C I, II, VI	☐ C III, VI, VIII	☐ C II, IV, V, VII
☐ D III, VI, VIII	☐ D I, IV, VI	☐ D I, II, VI
☐ E II, III, VII, VIII	☐ E II, III, VII, VIII	☐ E II, III, VII, VIII
☐ F I, VI, VII	☐ F V, VI, VIII	☐ F I, IV, VI
☐ G III, V, VII	☐ G II, IV, V, VII	☐ G V, VI, VIII
☐ H V, VI, VIII	☐ H I, II, VI	☐ H III, VI, VIII

Answers to Question 31 are on page 260

Chart One

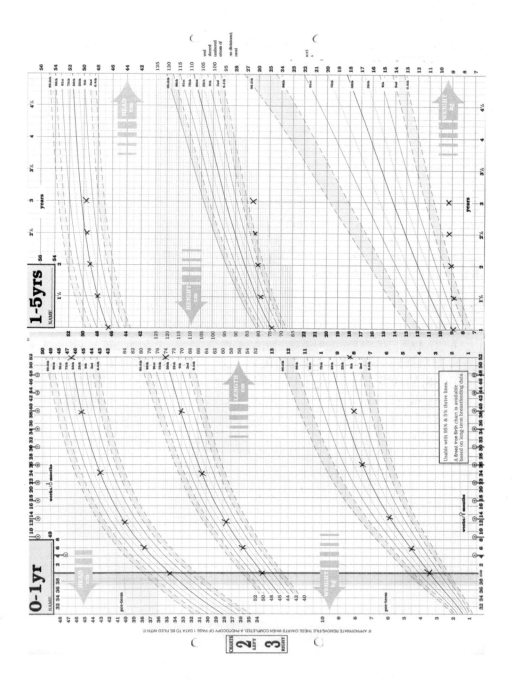

Chart Two

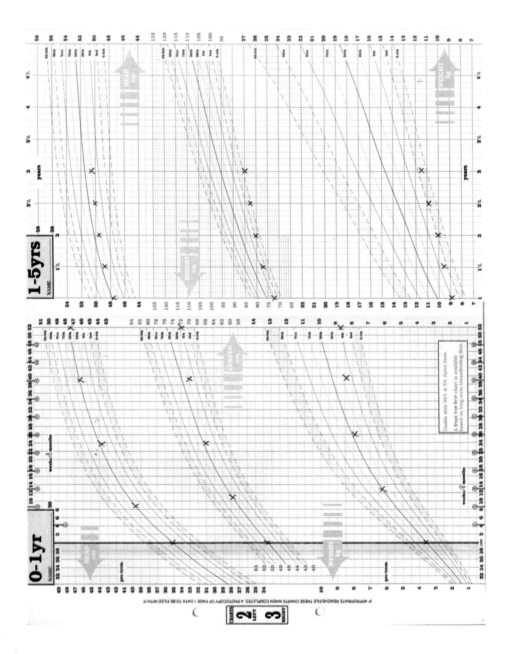

Chart Three

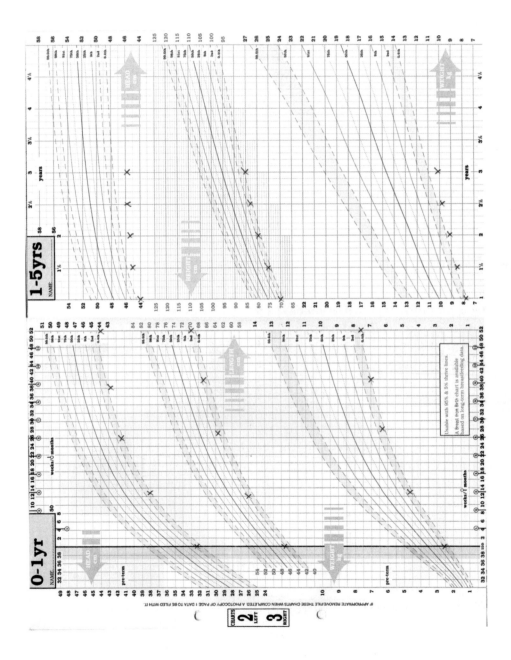

ANSWERS TO QUESTION 31

If an infant or young child experiences deceleration of a previously established growth pattern, or is growing at consistently below the 3rd centile, the pattern of growth of weight, height and head circumference can help establish a likely cause. The charts in this question illustrate the three main types of impaired growth:

Chart One

A I

Retardation of weight with near-normal or slowly decelerating height and head circumference. This pattern of growth is typically seen in undernutrition.

Chart Two

G II, IV, V, VII

Near-proportional retardation of weight and height with normal head circumference. This pattern of growth is typical of that found with constitutional growth delay, genetic short stature, endocrinopathies and skeletal dysplasia.

Chart Three:

H III, VI, VIII

Concomitant retardation of weight, height and head circumference. A pattern of growth typically associated with in utero and perinatal insults, chromosomal aberrations and CNS abnormalities. It may also (rarely) be familial.

QUESTION 32

A 5-day-old term baby is noted to be having abnormal movements by the midwifery team. He was born by elective lower segment caesarean section (ELSCS) for breech presentation. No resuscitation was required, and he was transferred to the postnatal wards with mother on day 1 of life. Feeding was established without major difficulty and first day check was normal.

The pregnancy history was unremarkable, mother's booking serology required no specific action and an anomaly scan was normal at 21 weeks' gestation. It was at that time he was first noted to be a breech presentation. The pregnancy proceeded uneventfully with apparently normal intrauterine growth. By 36 weeks' gestation he remained a breech presentation and so an attempt was made at external cephalic version, which was not successful. No fetal distress followed and ELSCS was at 39 weeks' gestation. His mother had a heavy cold the week of delivery.

The baby is reviewed on day 5 of life. He is feeding well and examination is normal. The diagnosis of benign myoclonus of infancy is made and he is discharged home for routine community follow up.

On day 10 of life he is rushed back into hospital by ambulance. He had been on mother's lap and had suddenly stopped breathing. He had then gone blue and stiff and developed jerking of one arm and one leg. When the ambulance crew arrived he looked 'well' but on the way to hospital he had a further similar episode. In A&E he is apyrexial, well perfused and neurological examination is normal. He is started on intravenous antibiotics and acyclovir and is admitted to the ward for further assessment.

His 3-year-old sister had a febrile seizure at 8 months of age but has been well since and is developing normally. There is no other family history of epilepsy or febrile seizures.

32.1 Which of the following would be an appropriate initial choice of antibiotic treatment?

☐ A Ceftriaxone
☐ B Benzylpenicillin and flucloxacillin
☐ C Benzylpenicillin and gentamicin
☐ D Cefuroxime and gentamicin
☐ E Vancomycin and gentamicin
☐ F Ceftazidime and gentamicin
☐ G Flucloxacillin and gentamicin
☐ H Ceftriaxone and amoxycillin

Initial investigations are as follows:

Haemoglobin:	14.7 g/dl
White cell count:	11×10^9/litre
Platelets:	212×10^9/litre
C-reactive protein:	6 mg/litre
Sodium:	141 mmol/litre
Potassium:	3.7 mmol/litre
Urea:	3.4 mmol/litre
Creatinine:	35 μmol/litre
Alanine transaminase:	32 IU/litre
Bilirubin:	49 μmol/litre
Albumin:	42 g/litre
Glucose:	5.1 mmol/litre
Calcium:	2.5 mmol/litre
Phosphate:	1.8 mmol/litre
Magnesium:	0.9 mmol/litre
Blood culture:	No growth after 48 hours
Urinary dipstix:	NAD
CSF:	

CSF:
    WBC: 8×10^6 cells/litre (80% polys)
    Protein: 0.5 g/litre
    Glucose: 3.6 mmol/litre
    No growth after 48 hours

An EEG is performed which is reported to be normal. He continues to have seizures several times a day. An EEG is performed again, this time while a seizure is occurring. The background activity is generally slow and in the clonic phase of the seizure generalised spike activity is noted. In between the seizures the baby remains very well and feeds well. In view of the regularity of the seizures, phenobarbitone is commenced and within 72 hours the seizures stop. He is discharged home 3 days later.

32.2 What is the most likely diagnosis?

- [ ] A Hypoxic ischaemic encephalopathy
- [ ] B Benign neonatal familial convulsion
- [ ] C Pyridoxine dependency
- [ ] D Herpes simplex encephalitis
- [ ] E Neonatal drug withdrawal
- [ ] F Munchausen syndrome by proxy

32.3 What will you advise the parents on the likelihood of their baby developing epilepsy in infancy and childhood?

- [ ] A 10%
- [ ] B 100%
- [ ] C 50%
- [ ] D Nil
- [ ] E It is not possible to estimate at this stage

32.4 Which ONE of the following would be most helpful?

- [ ] A CT head scan
- [ ] B Video EEG
- [ ] C Further detailed history
- [ ] D Urine toxicology screen
- [ ] E MRI scan brain
- [ ] F CSF PCR HSV
- [ ] G Trial of pyridoxine during EEG monitoring
- [ ] H Case conference

ANSWERS TO QUESTION 32

32.1 H   Ceftriaxone and amoxycillin
32.2 B   Benign neonatal familial convulsion
32.3 A   10%
32.4 C   Further detailed history

Discussion

In a neonate presenting with seizures, empirical treatment for presumed sepsis (meningo-encephalitis) is mandatory. In Question 32.1, 'H' is the only option that offers cover against all the likely causes of bacterial meningo-encephalitis in this age group. This combination will cover group B streptococcus, *Streptococcus pneumoniae,* Gram-negative organisms (eg *Escherichia coli, Klebsiella pneumoniae, Neisseria meningitidis, Haemophilus influenzae*) and *Listeria monocytogenes.* Amoxycillin is specifically included to provide cover against the latter.

The differential diagnosis offered in Question 32.2 is broad. There is nothing in the history to support a diagnosis of drug withdrawal. Bacterial meningitis is excluded by the CSF results. Herpes simplex encephalitis and non-accidental injury are both unlikely given that this baby is well between seizures and has normal CSF. An inborn error of metabolism is unlikely given that this baby is not persistently obtunded and has a normal glucose, bicarbonate, lactate, ammonia and ALT. Seizures occurring as a result of hypoxic ischaemic encephalopathy first occur typically within the first 48 hours of life and not for the first time at 10 days of age. Pyridoxine dependency should be considered when generalized seizures (typically resistant to phenobarbitone and phenytoin) begin soon after birth following signs of fetal distress in utero. Administration of 100–200 mg of pyridoxine to affected infants will abruptly terminate the seizures, with normalisation of the EEG within a few hours.

The most likely diagnosis in this case is benign neonatal familial convulsion. This is an autosomal dominant potassium channelopathy that occurs early in the neonatal period. Seizures may occur as frequently as 10–20 times per day, though affected neonates are typically well between seizures, as in this case (This child's father gave a clear history of being similarly affected during the neonatal period and early infancy.)

Phenobarbitone is an effective treatment and can usually be withdrawn after 6–9 months of age without relapse. The condition carries a 10% risk of ⊗ generalised seizures later in life (Surtees, 2000).

Reference

Surtees, R. 2000. Inherited ion channel disorders. *European Journal of Pediatrics* **159**(Suppl. 3): S199–203.

QUESTION 33

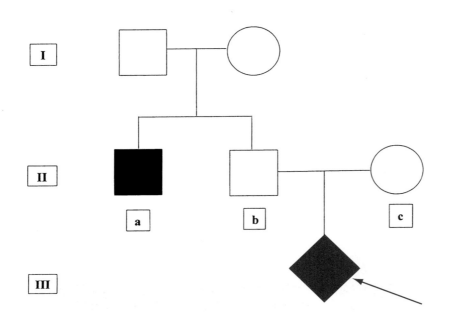

33.1   In the above karyotype IIa is affected with cystic fibrosis. What
       is the risk that the fetus indicated by the red diamond will also
       have the disease, assuming that both parents are healthy?

☐ A   1 in 2000
☐ B   1 in 20
☐ C   1 in 400
☐ D   1 in 30
☐ E   1 in 80
☐ F   1 in 120
☐ G   1 in 6
☐ H   1 in 4

Answers to Question 33 are on page 268

ANSWERS TO QUESTION 33

Cystic fibrosis is the most common autosomal recessive disorder in caucasians, with an incidence of 1 in 2000. 1 in 20 of the general population are carriers for this condition. In the family tree provided, since IIa is affected with the condition, both his parents must be carriers. The chance of his brother being a carrier is 2/3, since we are told in the question that he is not affected by CF. The chance of IIc being a carrier is 1/20, the population risk. The chance of this fetus having CF is therefore:

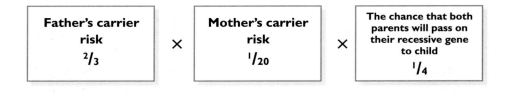

| Father's carrier risk $^2/_3$ | × | Mother's carrier risk $^1/_{20}$ | × | The chance that both parents will pass on their recessive gene to child $^1/_4$ |

$$= {}^1/_{120}$$

QUESTION 34

A 2-year-old boy is referred by his GP with a 2-day history of passing large, dark, extremely offensive, non-mucousy stools. He has not had diarrhoea or constipation, and there is no history of vomiting. He has complained of mild 'tummy pain' in the last few days and has lost his appetite. He is managing to sleep at night and on direct enquiry there are no other symptoms of note. Past medical history is unremarkable. He was born at term by spontaneous vaginal delivery and was well in the neonatal period. He has had normal developmental surveillance screening, has been fully immunised and he is not on any medication. His family are well.

On examination he is pale and lethargic but alert. Basic observations are temperature 37.2°C, heart rate 140, blood pressure 85/30 and respiratory rate 24. Cardiovascular and respiratory systems are otherwise normal. He is tender around the umbilicus but there is no organomegaly, palpable mass, rebound or guarding. A small anal fissure is noted around the anal margin. Bowel sounds are reduced. He passes a black, tarry highly offensive stool in the department in which there is also some fresh blood.

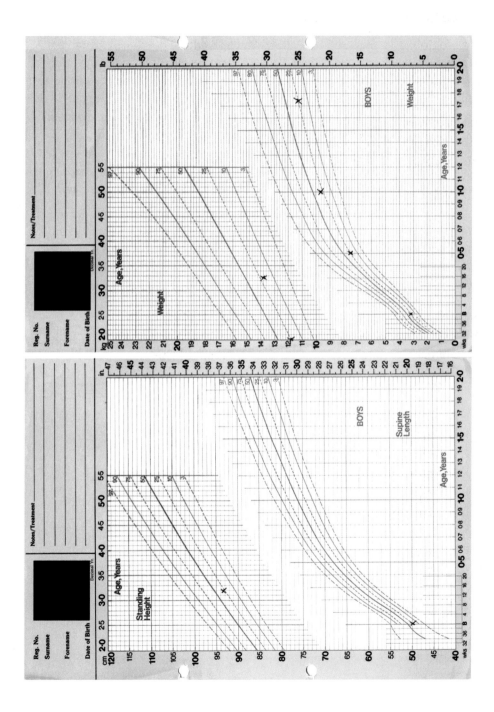

Initial investigations are as follows:

Haemoglobin:	5.9 g/dl
White cell count:	10.2×10^9/litre
Platelets:	158×10^9/litre
ESR:	22 mm/h
Prothrombin time:	13 seconds
Activated partial thromboplastin time:	32 seconds
Fibrinogen:	1.9 g/litre
Sodium:	138 mmol/litre
Potassium:	4.9 mmol/litre
Urea:	7.2 mmol/litre
Creatinine:	43 μmol/litre
CRP:	6 g/litre
Alanine transaminase:	45 IU/litre
Albumin:	36 g/litre
Bilirubin:	18 μmol/litre
Alkaline phosphatase:	178 IU/litre
Abdominal X-ray:	unremarkable

34.1 What is the most likely diagnosis?

- [ ] A Crohn's disease
- [ ] B Von Willebrand's disease
- [ ] C Haemolytic uraemic syndrome
- [ ] D Intussusception
- [ ] E Meckel's diverticulum
- [ ] F Ulcerative colitis
- [ ] G Gastrointestinal arteriovenous malformation
- [ ] H Duodenal ulceration
- [ ] I Bleeding from an anal fissure
- [ ] J Bacterial enteritis
- [ ] K Oesophageal varices

34.2 After initial resuscitation, which ONE of the following investigations would be most helpful in making the diagnosis?

- [ ] A Endoscopy
- [ ] B Blood film
- [ ] C Air enema
- [ ] D Technetium scintigraphy
- [ ] E Colonoscopy with biopsy of the colon
- [ ] F Detailed coagulation study
- [ ] G Proctoscopy
- [ ] H Stool culture
- [ ] I Barium enema

Answers to Question 34 are on page 274

ANSWERS TO QUESTION 34

34.1 E   Meckel's diverticulum
34.2 D   Technetium scintigraphy

Discussion

This child presented with painless melaena, for which the commonest cause at this age is bleeding associated with a Meckel's diverticulum. Intussusception is an important differential diagnosis. In this case melaena or partially altered blood, in the absence of vomiting, significant abdominal pain, a palpable mass and with an unremarkable abdominal X-ray, collectively mediate against the diagnosis of intussusception. Melaena is not typical in haemolytic uraemic syndrome, and one would expect a clearer history of gastroenteritis if this were a likely diagnosis. The short history, normal growth, albumin and platelet count, with near-normal inflammatory markers make inflammatory bowel disease very unlikely. The normal clotting profile in part mediates against Von Willebrand's disease, and portal hypertension with secondary oesophageal varices is not supported by the normal PT and liver function tests. Bleeding from an upper gastrointestinal arteriovenous malformation or from duodenal ulceration are both theoretically possible, but as the question asks for the most likely underlying diagnosis, Meckel's diverticulum is the preferred answer.

Meckel's diverticulum occurs in 2% of all infants and symptoms usually present in the first 2 years of life. The acid-secreting ectopic mucosa, which lines the diverticulum, causes ulceration of the normal adjacent ileal mucosa with consequent bleeding and often anaemia, as in this case. Less common manifestations include bowel obstruction, which may occur when the diverticulum acts a lead point for an intussusception, and acute diverticulitis which may mimic acute appendicitis.

In a 'Meckel's scan' technetium is taken up by mucus-secreting cells of the ectopic gastric mucosa, facilitating visualisation of the diverticulum. Scan sensitivity is as high as 85% when uptake is enhanced by cimetidine or glucagon, and specificity of the order of 95%. Surgical excision is curative.

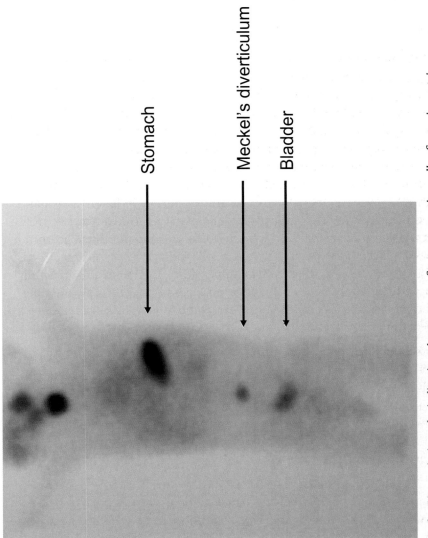

Stomach

Meckel's diverticulum

Bladder

Technetium scintigraphy indicating the presence of mucus-secreting cells of ectopic gastric mucosa within a Meckel's diverticulum

INDEX